INTRA-ARTICULAR
I N J E C T I O N S

INTRA-ARTICULAR INJECTIONS

SECOND EDITION

Sureshwar Pandey
MBBS (Hons) MS (Gen) FICS FIAMS MS (Ortho) FACFAC FACS FNAMS
Professor Emeritus University of Ranchi
Founder and Founder Director GNH Handicapped Children Hospital and RJS Artificial Limb Centre
Founder and Consultant Ram Janam Sulakshana Institute of Orthopaedics and Research, Ranchi.
Founder and Founder President and Sec. General Indian Foot Society (Affiliated to International Federation of Foot and Ankle Societies IFFAS).
Founder and Emeritus Editor: The Journal of Foot Surgery
Visiting Professor: Universities of Tokyo, Osaka, Teikyo, Adelaide, Flienders, Vjung Pandang, Singapore
ex-Chairman ASIA-CIP (IFFAS)
Founder and Chairman Ram Janam Sulakshana Pandey Cancer Hospital and Research and Rehabilitation Centre, Ranchi

Anil Kumar Pandey
MBBS, CORM, Ph.D Orth, MAMS
Director and Consultant
Ram Janam Sulakshana Institute of Orthopaedics and Research (RJSIOR), Ranchi
Asst. Director and Consultant
GNH Handicapped Children Hospital and RJS Artificial Limb Centre, Ranchi
Consultant Ram Janam Sulakshana Pandey Cancer Hospital and Research and Rehabilitation Centre, Ranchi

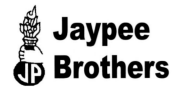
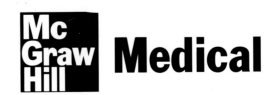

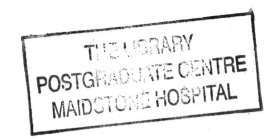
First published in India by

Jaypee Brothers Medical Publishers (P) Ltd
EMCA House, 23/23B Ansari Road, Daryaganj, New Delhi 110 002, India
Phones: +91-11-23272143, +91-11-23272703, +91-11-23282021, +91-11-23245672
Fax: +91-11-23276490, +91-11-23245683   e-mail: jaypee@jaypeebrothers.com
Visit our website: www.jaypeebrothers.com

First published in USA by The McGraw-Hill Companies, 2 Penn Plaza, New York, NY 10121-2298. Exclusively worldwide distributor except South Asia (India, Nepal, Sri Lanka, Bhutan, Pakistan, Bangladesh).

NOTICE

Medicine is an ever-changing science. As new research and clinical experience broaden our knowledge, changes in treatment and drug therapy are required. The authors and the publisher of this work have checked with sources believed to be reliable in their efforts to provide information that is complete and generally in accord with the standards accepted at the time of publication. However, in view of the possibility of human error changes in medical science, neither the editors nor the publisher nor any other party who has been involved in the preparation or publication of this work warrants that the information contained herein is in every respect accurate or complete, and they disclaim all responsibility for any errors or omissions or for the results obtained from use of the information contained in this work. Readers are encouraged to confirm the information contained herein with other sources. For example and in particular, readers are advised to check the product information sheet included in the package of each drug they plan to administer to be certain that the information contained in this work is accurate and that changes have not been made in the recommended dose or in the contraindications for administration. This recommendation is of particular importance in connection with new or infrequently used drugs.

ISBN   0-07-148582-1
ISBN 13 9780071485821

to
the fond memory of my beloved parents
Sulakshana Pandey
and
Ramjanam Pandey
who were, are, and will be
always with me to love, teach and guide
who taught me to persue my
dreams—because nothing is impossible

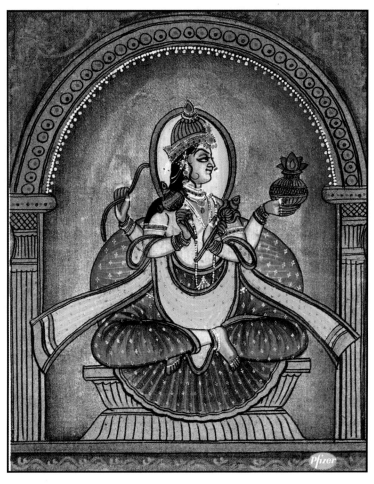

"DHANVANTARI"*
The Hindu God of Medicine

Commonly worshipped as the Hindu God of Medicine, DHANVANTARI is regarded as the original exponent of Indian medicine. DHANVANTARI has many myths and legends woven around him. He emerged with the pot of ambrosia (symbolic of medicine) in his hand from the ocean when it was churned by the contesting gods and demons. He is viewed as the very incarnation of God VISHNU. He is said to have recovered ambrosia which had been lost, and thus obtained a share in sacrifices.

Legends make him reappear as "DIVODASA", the prince of Benaras (Kasiraja), in the family of Ayus. Dhanvantari, Divodasa and Kasiraja are names of the same person who is "the first god and who freed the other gods from old age, disease and death", and who in his Himalayan retreat

---

* This painting has been commissioned by Pfizer Ltd (India) based on an old painting belonging to the Late Maharaja of Mysore, Krishnaraja Wodeyar II (South India).

taught surgery to Susruta and other sages. DHANVANTARI appeared on earth in Benaras in the princely family of Bahuja and became known as Divodasa; he wandered about as a mendicant even during his early years.

DHANVANTARI also appears to have been an actual historical person, although his precise identity is hard to be ascertained. He taught surgery and other divisions of Ayurveda (Indian system of medicine) at the instance of Susruta, to a group of sages among whom Susruta was the foremost. DHANVANTARI is regarded as the patron-God of all branches of medicine. While DHANVANTARI is not credited with any medical treatise of his own, in the early accounts, there is a voluminous glossary and materia medica in the nine sections known as Dhanvantari-Nighantu; it is a compilation which is probably contemporaneous with the famous Amara-kosha (A.D. 100). There are a few other works which are also ascribed to Dhanvantari.

There are numerous preparations which are ascribed to him, and many of them quite ancient.

Dhanvantari-Nighantu is considered the most ancient of the medical glossaries that are available. The original work is said to have been in three recensions; the present version which may have been based on one of them, is in six sections and deals with 373 medicinal substances; their names, synonyms, and brief description of properties being given. The work which claims to be 'like the third eye' for the practising physician, is extensively relied upon, despite several more comprehensive glossaries that have been compiled subsquently. Since there is no authentic source of information, this text can be considered more as indicative.

(By courtesy Pfizer Limited)

Acknowledgements

It is always difficult to organise and sustain academic activity especially in print format, but for the doggedness and sustained enthusiasm, which only gets augmented by the observations over the subjects—the patients. We are obliged to them for providing experiences to us to the extent which stimulated us to bring out the Second Edition.

Unless the users—the young orthopaedic and general surgeons, rheumatologists and even general practitioners—would have accepted the First Edition willingly, the stimulus to bring out the Second Edition would not have been sustained. We are indebted to them.

Arranging the manuscript and putting them in proper order and further printing it out are really great annoying jobs. These all have been very gladly and patiently done by my dear grand-daughter Pallavi and dear Secretary Sheeja. I (SP) cannot return their debt.

My (SP's) grandchildren—Pallavi, Shivam, Vaishnavi, Shruti, Soumya and Satyam have been real source of easing tension of my life with pleasant moments with them—God bless them always.

I bow my head to the feet of my Revd. illustrious fatherly teacher Padma Bhushan Emeritus Professor B. Mukhopadhaya, who remained the perennial source of inspiration for me.

How can I forget the immense help of Shri JP Vij, the CMD of Jaypee Brothers Medical Publishers (P) Ltd, and all persons involved in producing such a nice monograph. We are really thankful to one and all of Jaypee Brothers.

Contents

CHAPTER 1

Principles of Intra-articular and Allied Injections

INTRODUCTION

It is more than five decades from now that Philip Hench and his colleagues introduced the corticosteroids with a lot of fan and fair (triumphal and trumpeted introduction indeed) for managing rheumatoid arthritis at the Mayo clinic in 1949.

In fact Kendall and Hench in America and Reichstein in Switzerland jointly won the Nobel Prize for the introduction of cortisone, which was used for the first time in 1948 for treating rheumatoid arthritis. Soon after it was observed by Philip Hench and his colleagues at Mayo clinic (1949) that hydrocortisone was active at tissue level in reducing the inflammatory changes. However now responsible physicians always want to ward off the steroids or wean them off (if it has already being used) as far as possible. Of course, its one use still remains and perhaps will remain (till some harmless substitute come in the medical arena) universally employed and that is its intra-articular, periarticular and intra-lesional injections/infiltrations.

Joe Hollander (1951) was the first to introduce its local infiltrative use to control pain and limit the inflammatory process, whether induced by trauma, collagen arthropathy or crystallopathy or similar conditions. Oral use of corticosteroids is very popular with the physicians even general practitioners, but its local use demands a skilled approach, a knowledge placement and careful precautions to avoid infections. The surgeons or rheumatologists or gynaecologists or dermatologists or ophthalmologists need to know absolutely where, when, how, why and why not to use it.

Hollander was perhaps one of the first to use compound F (hydrocortisone acetate) into an inflamed joint due to rheumatoid arthritis, and had also used prednisolone tertiary butyl acetate to prolong the benefit. Hydrocortisone acetate (an acetate ester of hydrocortisone) is a very fine white odourless crystalline powder and is practically insoluble in water (considerably less soluble than the hydrocortisone in aqueous media). It melts at a temperature of 216-220°C. One gram dissolves in 230 ml of alcohol and 150 ml of chloroform.

The preparation most commonly effectively and widely used till recently is hydrocortisone tertiary acetate ester of triamcinolone acetinide (TATBA). The chemical formula of hydrocortisone acetate is $C_{23}H_{32}O_6$. The injection available is a sterile suspension of hydrocortisone acetate in sodium chloride solution, containing a dispersing agent.

The usual dose of hydrocortisone acetate for intra-articular injection is 25 mg for an average joint with a variation from 0.5 to 50 mg. Several joints can be injected simultaneously.

MODE OF ACTION

Glucocorticoids diffuse across the cell membrane and form a complex with specific cytoplasmic receptors. These complexes enter the nucleus of the cell, bind to the DNA and stimulate transcription of mRNA, and later protein synthesis of various enzymes. On the whole, this is the basic biochemical action of the steroid which accounts for the various and numerous effects after the systemic use.

As such the mode of action of adrenocortical steroids has been mainly discussed around:

1. Immune responses
2. Anti-inflammatory properties

However they also influence the carbohydrate, protein and fat metabolism. They also affect the working of cardiovascular system, skeletal system, skeletal muscles and the central nervous system.

IMMUNE RESPONSES

The mode of immune responses, as yet, has not been clearly defined. They are believed to modify the clinical course of different diseases in which hypersensitivity is believed to play an important role. They do not interfere with the normal mechanism of development of cell-mediated immunity. Probably, they prevent or suppress the inflammatory responses that take place as a consequence of hypersensitivity reactions.

ANTI-INFLAMMATORY PROPERTIES

Researches are still on to understand clearly the anti-inflammatory properties of corticoids. However for the clinicians it is perhaps enough to understand that corticoids inhibit the inflammatory responses, whether the inciting agent is radiant, mechanical, chemical, infectious or immunological. It must be borne in mind that there is only suppression of the inflammatory effect, while the underlying causes of the diseases remain unaffected. It is this property of corticoids that provides them almost unique potential for therapeutic disaster. Hence, the epitomized remark, at times, stands true that corticoids, if misused, permit a patient to walk slowly all the way to the autopsy room. However, the recent works in more detail have projected variable positive thinking about the role of intra-articular corticosteroids.

Corticosteroids exert their anti-inflammatory action by interrupting the inflammatory and immune cascade at several levels including: impairment of antigen opsonisation, interference with inflammatory cell adhesion and migration through vascular endothelium, interruption of cell-cell communication by alteration of release or antagonism of cytokines (interleukin –1), impairment of leukotriene and prostaglandin synthesis, inhibition of production of neutrophil superoxide, metalloprotease and metalloprotease activator (plasminogen activator), and decreased immunoglobulin synthesis (Gaffney et al 1995).

Against earlier reported that corticosteroids injections may suppress cartilage proteoglycan synthesis, worsen cartilage lesion, or even cause degenerative lesion in normal cartilage (Raynauld 1999), recent reports have shown that low dose intra-articular corticosteroids (sufficient to suppress catabolism) normalised proteoglycan synthesis and significantly reduced the incidence and severity of cartilage erosions and osteophyte formation (Raynauld JP et al, 2003). In humans, repeated corticosteroid injection in knees of patients with chronic arthritis presented no evidence of destruction or accelerated deterioration (Friedman and Moore 1980).

The local or intra-articular injection of the corticoids does not appear to have significant systemic effects. However, it does not mean that it is all full proof. Slowly there may be a gross damage of the articular cartilage following injudiceous repeated use of intra-articular corticoids.

The local mode of action is again not clearly defined. Though pioneers have devoted their time and mind to illustrate the exact mode of action of intra-articular hydrocortisone acetate and allied substance (Table 1 on page 81) the controversy still exists. Kantrowitz et al (1975) suggested that the anti-inflammatory property of corticosteroid emanate from their capacity to inhibit production of prostaglandin (a potent mediator of inflammatory response) in the synovium.

Clinical effects of suppression of non-specific inflammation and reduction of swelling and pain to varying extent have been noticed in most of the cases with intra-articular injection of the corticosteroids. However, in certain cases it appears as only a pallative therapy and at another few occasions it proves to be ineffective.

It has been noticed that at times even a placebo injection into the joint or even just pricking into the joint helps in relieving the chronic pain to varying extent. This may be explained, more or less on the comparable lines of using electrical stimulation and acupuncture to relieve the chronic pain.

Probably, they act by closing a hypothetical GATE in the spinal cord, thereby blocking pain stimuli from reaching the brain. Puncturing stimulates small nerve fibres sending impulses through the OPEN GATE that registers in brain as acute pain. When the signals reach the central biasing mechanism of the brainstem, they trigger counter impulses, which travel down the spinal cord and close the GATE against the chronic pain. However, this is just a hypothesis. Various research works, being done to find the effective ways and means of tackling the problem of pain, point to a new attractive approach basing upon the opposite principles of stimulating the inhibitory systems. Of course it is too early to provide an objective evaluation of such possibilities. Low doses of intra-articular steroids have been noticed to reduce the size, severity and progression of both, lesions of the cartilage and osteophyte formation (William 1985, Pelletier et al 1994).

Though Moskowitz et al (1985) and Behrens (1975) have raised the possibilities of adverse effects of intra-articular corticosteroids on the articular cartilage, varying benefits from such injections cannot be denied (Freidman 1980, Dieppe et al 1980, Pandey 1982), rather its judicious use can always be beneficial (Pandey 1982).

It has been general tendency to use intra-articular steroids in late stage of osteoarthritis or other similar arthritic conditions, but this strategy needs to be changed in light of the experimental evidences, which indicate that intra-articular steroids exert a chondro-protective effect—it is probably by the suppression of stromelysin synthesis, a metalloprotease implicated in osteoarthritic cartilage degradation. However, though pain relief by intra-articular corticosteroids can be dramatic, its long-term chondroprotective effects need further authentication.

Hydrocortisone the natural hormone, being too much soluble was found to disperse too quickly and thus could not leave its prolonged effects locally. Hence, its chemically improved ester form hydrocortisone acetate ($C_{23}H_{32}O_6$) the primary alcohol group of C_{23} being the one esterified was developed and found to be suitable. It is considerably less soluble than hydrocortisone in aqueous media, rather for all practical purposes hydrocortisone acetate may be taken as insoluble in water. It melts at a temperature of 216–220°C. One gram dissolves in 230 ml of alcohol and 150 ml of chloroform. When prepared in microcrystalline form and mixed with other agents it forms a stable suspension, which can be injected locally where it remains deposited for several weeks, gradually releasing the hydrocortisone to produce its anti-inflammatory effects for longer period. The successful attempt to restore the comfort and mobility of rheumatoid affected joints by local injection of hydrocortisone acetate (compound F) into the inflamed joint was by Hollander, the Philadelphia rheumatologist in 1951. He used prednisolone tertiary butyl acetate to prolong the benefit. Mc Carty, the Hollander's colleague rheumatologist in Philadelphia, showed that the very long lasting synthetic corticosteroid derivatives, especially triamcinolone hexacetonide (TATBA or THA), could produce remarkable and lasting remissions of the rheumatoid arthritis effects when given as multiple injections at certain intervals, especially in smaller joints (e.g in hands). He equated the result to the 'medical synovectomy'. With the pioneering work of these two rheumatologists ushered the art and science of local injection therapy for the rheumatic disorders. Of course, the experiences of ameliorating pain by injecting local anaesthetic agents into and around the painful spots in the muscles and painful ligaments in the sprains have definite role in establishing the local injection therapy for rheumatoid disorders and allied conditions.

Gradually, there has been great swing in favour of injecting methylprednisolone acetate (chemical name being 6-methyl-delta-1-hydrocortisone) in place of hydrocortisone acetate, wherever it is indicated. It is 6-methyl derivative of prednisolone. Methylprednisolone acetate posses the general properties of the glucocorticoid methylprednisolone, but is less soluble and therefore less readily metabolized. Thus, after injection into various sites its action is prolonged. It is more or less white odourless crystalline powder which melts at about 215 degree C. with slight decomposition and is practically insoluble in water. Its molecular formula is "$C_{22}H_{30}O_5$" and has the molecular weight of 374.46.

Like other glucocorticoids, methylprednisolone causes profound and varied metabolic effects. These compounds have also been seen to modify the body's immune response to diverse stimuli.

POTENCY

The potency of 4 mg of methylprednisolone can be obtained from 4.4 mg of methylprednisolone acetate. The anti-inflammatory effect of 20 mg of hydrocortisone is available from the 4.4 mg of methylprednisolone acetate. Mineralocorticoid activity of methylprednisolone is minimal. 200 mg of methylprednisolone is equivalent to 1 mg of desoxycorticosterone. Intra-articular injection of Dysprosium-165-ferric hydroxide macroaggregates has been used for medical synovectomy, and has been proved to be an effective treatment for chronic rheumatoid synovitis of the knee with minimum radiographic evidence of lesion of bone and cartilage (stage I or stage II radiographic changes).

The low rates of systemic spread of the istope offer a definite advantage over previously used agents for radiation synovectomy, e.g. chemical such as osmic acid and alkylating agents, e.g (thiotepa and nitrogen mustard); several radionuclides in colloidal or particulate form, e.g. yttrium-90, gold-198, ebrium-169, rhenium-186, and phosphorus-32 (Sledge et al 1987). Dysphrosium-165 is a rare earth element with a half-life of 2.3 hours. It decays mainly by beta emissions. The maximum extent of penetration of the beta emission into the soft tissue is 5.7 millimetres, which probably approximates the entire synovial lining of the joint.

CHAPTER 2

How Frequently to Inject?

In case of hydrocortisone acetate, since the preparation used is in acetate form of suspension, there has to be slow dispersal of the drug. It is rather difficult to pin point the number of injections required for a particular case, but a working line can be projected on the basis of experiences.

Probably, the most suitable schedule will be at three weeks intervals and never to be repeated in less than two weeks. Even the intervals of 4 to 6 weeks has been found to be equally suitable and effective in several instances. Hence the working rule should be to keep an interval of not less than two weeks and not more than six weeks. It has been observed that if three consecutive injections are not effective in ameliorating the patients condition to appreciable extent, it will be probably not effective even with more injections. In such conditions, considering the possible hazards of intra-articular hydrocortisone acetate injections it should be abandoned henceforth. In giving bi-weekly injections, the moment symptoms are completely relieved, no further injection should be given. Even if the symptoms are not completely relieved upto five, weekly or fortnightly, injections, further injection should not be given. It has been observed that the cases which are going to respond, usually show adequate response at the very first properly given injection. If there is no appreciable response when injection into the synovial space is given as determined by the aspiration of synovial fluid, repeated injections may be futile, rather may be even harmful. The interval between two pricks may be placed between two to four weeks. Perhaps, beyond four weeks, relief obtained after the first injection may not be adequately carried over. Of course, in certain circumstances where, per chance, arthrotomy happened to be performed even after several months of intra-articular injections, the chalky deposits of hydrocortisone acetate could be demonstrated at different places in the joint, specially near about the attachments of intra-articular ligaments (e.g. cruciate ligament in knee, ligamentum teres in head and femur) or at the margins of capsular attachment.

James et al (1996) observed that in most patients of osteoarthritis, corticoid injections provide pain relief but it may not last for more than a few weeks. However, this observation is true in very less number of cases, rather many remain pain-free for more longer period (several months to year or even more sometimes).

Why Should Intra-articular Corticoid not be given More Frequently?

Perhaps there is hardly any general toxicity of local corticoid injections, but the local damaging effects over the structures of the joints have been noticed. Neuropathic-like changes on the structures of the joints especially in the knee (most frequent site of intra-articular injection of corticoids) have been reported. Whether the changes are subsequent to prolonged repeated injections of local anesthetics or local injection of corticoid or both, is matter of controversy. However, adequate experimental evidences have been gathered to blame corticoid injections to be responsible for neuropathic like changes in the joints.

The overall economic factor should also not be ignored as patients have to come from varying distance to proper place for intra-articular injections. In such circumstances, there does not appear any logic in asking the patient to come repeatedly if the initial response is not adequate. In the absence of early adequate response the patient should not be kept hanging on wishful thinkings. Rather than repeating intra-articular corticoid injection the surgeon should resort to appropriate surgical intervention.

Whether Intra-articular Corticoid should be Given as Cocktail or Alone?

In joints having easily definable space, corticoid may be injected alone. However, a cocktail of corticoid, lidocaine hydrochloride and hyaluronidase have been advocated to be more effective, when it is to be given in the soft tissues rather than into the synovial spaces. The hyaluronidase undoubtedly helps in easily spreading the corticosteroid. It seems to have no other advantage. However, it is a foreign protein, and allergy may develop if the injections are repeated, and it should be omitted in repeated use.

Hyaluronidase is a naturally occurring enzyme. It is found in the human (and mammals) semen, snake venom and certain bacteria. For clinical use it is purified so as to remove most of the inert material. The resultant solution is sterilized and freeze-dried into a white or yellowish white powder.

It has a temporary and reversible depolymerising action on the hyaluronic acid and chondroitin sulphate polysaccharides, which are normally present in the intercellular matrix of connective tissues. The intercellular cement is thus broken down thereby reducing its viscocity and rendering the tissues more permeable, which facilitates in rapid dispersal of the adjoining solution (e.g local anaesthetic, corticoid solution, transfusion fluid etc). It also promotes the reabsorption of excess fluid and blood from the tissues.

Hyaluronidase has been widely used in various fields (especially as an adjuvant to local anaesthetic agents) such as obstetric, ophthalmology, dentistry, anorectal and plastic surgery. In orthopaedics its use has been very limited (e.g for ganglion aspiration).

The standard dose is 1500 units of hyaluronidase injection.

The lidocaine is for local analgesia. In such circumstances the volume of injections should also be taken care of and the cocktail must be accordingly adjusted.

The joints like metacarpo-phalangeal, interphalangeal and temporomandibular ones, only hydrocortisone or other corticoids may be injected. But 0.5 to 1 ml of local anaesthetic may be added to act as a vehicle for smaller amount of drug. This also acts as local anaesthetic to some extent.

In joint, where surface area is more tortuous or intervened with more watershades e.g shoulder, hip and spinal joints, the cocktail of local anaesthetic and corticoid is suitable. It has been the practice in a few hands to infiltrate a local anaesthetic first, and to leave the needle there in the space. Subsequently the cocktail or corticoid alone is pushed into. This procedure is not always needed except for the beginners where the joint space may not be reached in a single direct prick. It carries a potential drawback that the joint space is communicating to be exterior threatening to carry the airborne infecting agents into the joints. Further manipulating the top of the open needle-end with bare fingers also carries the potential risk of contamination. Hence, wherever desired, it is better to prepare a cocktail earlier, load into the syringe and push directly into the desired space. The pain of prick will be always there, even for infiltrating the local anaesthetic prior to injecting the corticoid.

Many other preparations have been injected into the joints (See Table 1 on page 81). Others, which are essentially radioactive or chemical cauterising agents, are of limited specialised value and require special facilities and expertise.

Substances such as orgotein (pharmaceutical form of the bovine enzyme Cu-Zn superoxide dismutase), radiation synovectomy (dysprosium-165 hydroxide macroaggregate, yttrium–90 silicate), dextrose prolotherapy, silicone, saline lavage, saline injection without lavage, analgesic agents (bupivicaine, morphine), NSAIDs (tenoxicam, indoprofen, phenylbutazone, glucosamine, somatostatin, sodium pentosan polysulfate (NAPP), chloroquin, mucopolysaccharide polysulfuric acid ester, lactic acid solution, 10% dextrose, cytostatica (thiotepa, azetepa, osmium acid) have been investigated as potentially therapeutic in the treatment of arthritic joints.

CHAPTER 3

How to Inject?

Perhaps no one can predict in which particular case corticoid (or substitute) is going to provide relief, but everyone must take it for granted that even a slight negligence on the part of the injecting hand can spoil the joint for years or even forever.

Before injecting ask yourself a few questions:
- Does this joint require any injection into it?
- Is the surface over and around the joints free from infective focus?
- Are you competent enough to invade into the virginity of the joint?
- Is your patient free from diabetes?
- Are the syringe, needle and other equipments/instruments thoroughly sterilised?

WORD OF CAUTION

Let us be very honest, it is not certain in most of the cases where we are injecting hydrocortisone acetate or other steroids that we are definitely going to give relief to the patient but it is almost certain that we can always be culprit of introducing infective organism with devastating effects, perhaps irreversible in most of the cases, unless we are truly aseptic in our procedure. Let us not rob the patient of the residual utility of his joints, only with an uncertain attempt to suppress his painful stimuli. This does not mean that one should stop the corticoid injection, rather one must use it but with a flash of caution before every prick.

LOCALISATION OF THE SITE OF THE INJECTION

Since the point of injection must not be touched after cleaning, it is always essential to mark the injection spot prior to cleaning. Except for the bigger joint (e.g. knee, where joint line can be delineated easily at the either side of the ligamentum patellae) it is better to pinpoint the injection spot by prior marking. It is further important while injecting into soft tissue, e.g. for lateral epicondylitis, golfer's elbow.

Two methods can be adopted. Using the skin pencil, the joint line/or the point of maximum tenderness can be marked by cross point. Or thumbnail can be used to pinpoint the spot, by producing a dent, which remains visible even after washing and cleaning the area for injecting.

A reference point can also be selected which can be palpated by clean index fingertip, and the needle can be pushed at the nearby previously selected spot in relation to the reference point which is NOT touched at all after thorough cleaning—e.g. in knee joint, index finger tip of left hand can be placed in the infrapatellar fossa on lateral side, if injection has to be given through medial infrapatellar fossa or visa-versa. Similarly by locating the posterior angle of acromian process, the shoulder joint can be injected through a point just inferior to it without touching it.

CHAPTER 4

Indications

It has become a very common fashion to prescribe intra or periarticular or intra/peri-tendinous injections of corticoids. We may not be blamed for the statement that in conditions where we are not able to assign any specific cause, and especially if we are not able to allay the patient of the pain corticoid becomes an important feature of our prescription. Should we label it as a non-specific chemotherapeutic agent for such conditions? This version has a base, because in several non-specific painful conditions, corticoid infiltration does work. Patients get relieved of the symptoms, while the proper ailment remains undiagnosed. However, there are definite indications for its infiltrations. At several places it is used empirically and at frequent occasions it is a 'hit and miss' prescription.

Local corticoid therapy is a very precious therapeutic aid in rheumatology. Awareness and respect of its indications, contraindications and risks by the clinicians lead to very successful use of local corticoids in optimal conditions with minimal complications. However, in rheumatoid arthritis concurrent medical management accelerate the recovery. When the systemic gold therapy is contemplated even then local/intra-articular corticoid therapy should be considered.

Clear indications for intra-articular injection have not been charted out. However, workable indications may be put as follows:

DEFINITE INDICATIONS OF CORTICOID INJECTION

Convenient sites for intra-articular injection are the knee, ankle, wrist, elbow, shoulder, phalangeal, sternoclavicular and acromioclavicular joints. Difficulty is experienced in injecting into the hip joint. Anatomically inaccessible joints, such as spinal joints, and the joints devoid of synovial space, e.g. sacroiliac joints are not suitable for intra-articular injections.

1. Degenerative arthrosis of joint—primary or secondary.

2. Rheumatoid arthritis of joints—usually as an adjuvant to other appropriate medical and physical management.
3. Psoriatic arthropathy.
4. Peripheral synovial swelling of ankylosing spondylitis and of Reiter's syndrome.
5. Synovial structures (e.g. in joints, tendon, sheathes, bursae) are definite target, where local injection therapy prove useful. However, it should be avoided in uric acid gout, for which more effective treatments are available. Of course in acute gouty arthritis it has been found to be useful.
6. Post-traumatic stiffness of the joint.
7. Post-immobilization stiffness of the joint.
8. Periarthritis shoulder.
9. Non-specific fibrous ankylosis.
10. Intra-articular fractures—after aspiration of haemarthrosis—injection should be given—cautiously and only once.
11. Extra-articular tennis-elbow (lateral epicondylitis of humerus).
12. Golfer's-elbow (medial epicondylitis of humerus).
13. De-Quervain's disease.
14. Apophysitis e.g. Osgood-Schlatter disease, calcaneal apophysitis.

While targeting to inject certain zone/structure or/joint, there may be flowing of the injected fluid into the communicating pouches or sheaths or elsewhere. Sometimes there are naturally occurring communications such as those often found between the ankle joint and neighbouring tendon sheaths. Sometimes adventitious communications exist such as those developed in the shoulder region e.g. in rheumatoid arthritis when the gleno-humeral joint and subacromial bursae join together. At times synovial cysts develop near joints, where the communication is usually valvular, when the injected material flows into the synovial cyst but the reverse is not true. In these conditions too, other conservative methods of treatment must be exhausted earlier. In degenerative arthritis especially that of knee, there is definitive role of intra-articular corticoids injection. Other intra-articular substances such as orgetein, radiation synovectomy, dextrose prolotherapy, silicone, saline lavage, saline injection without lavage, analgesic agents, non-steroidal anti-inflammatory drugs, glucosamine, somatostatin, sodium pentosan polysulphate, chloroquine, mucopolysaccharide polysulphuric acid ester, lactic acid solution and thiotepa cytostatica have been tried as potentially therapeutic agent in the treatment of osteoarthritic joints. Recent observations have indicated that in primary osteoarthritis of knee, intra-articular Hylan G-F$_{20}$ treatment is effective for pain, disability and functional capacity. Low dose of intra-articular steroids reduce the size, severity and progression of both lesions of the cartilage and osteophyte formation (Williams 1985, Pelletier et al 1994). Even though there are possibilities of adverse effects on articular cartilage after repeated injections, its judicious use is mostly beneficial.

The strategy to use intra-articular steroids in late stages of osteoarthritis should be changed in the light of recent experimental evidences, which indicates that intra-articular steroids exert a chondro-protective effect probably by suppression of stromelysin synthesis—a metalloprotease implicated in osteoarthritic cartilage degradation (Pelletier 1989). However, though pain relief by intra-articular steroids can be dramatic its long-term chondroprotective effects need further authentification.

The overall review of the medical literature reflects that, in osteoarthritis corticosteroids and hyaluronic acid are widely used in patients who have not responded to other theraputic modalities. As a practical approach for a joint (like knee) with effusion, steroid injection should be considered, while in symptomatic dry joint hyaluronic acid approach should be useful.

RELATIVE INDICATIONS

Conditions have to be picked out from the list given below depending upon the earlier response to other available theraputic and conservative methods.

TENDONS (Mostly around and cautiously and very rarely into the tendons)

The objective is to bathe the tendon not to infiltrate it.

i. Tenosynovitis
ii. Peri-tendinitis
iii. Tendinitis (not more than two injections, since tendons are liable to rupture after repeated injections).
iv. Post-traumatic adhesions in and around tendons.
v. Ganglion in relation to tendon.
vi. Tendon involvement in collagen disorders.
vii. Post-operative tendon repair
   • To avoid adhesions—one or two injections only.
viii. Reconstruction or substitution of tendon.
ix. Early xanthomatous affection of tendon.
   • To hasten the recovery from pain and other effects on the joint due to immobilization and/ or operation (e.g. plaster cast, traction, arthroplasty).

LIGAMENTS

In most of the places where joint is infiltrated, ligaments (coming in the way) are also infiltrated but at places they may require specific infiltrations, e.g.

1. Partial avulsion of ligaments leading to pain.
2. Pellegrini Stieda disease.
3. Strained or sprained ligaments of a joint.
4. Post-traumatic adhesions of the ligaments.
5. Fibrotic nodule in relation to a ligament.
6. Collagen disorder affecting the ligaments.
7. Non-specific inflammation of the ligaments (e.g. plantar fascitis).

FIBROFATTY NODULES

Fibro-fatty nodules in relation to or even quite distant from the joint have been blamed as a triggering point for some painful conditions (sometimes quite unexplainable). In many cases they do respond to corticoid infiltration.

PERIPHERAL NERVES

Empirically along (perinural zone/sheath and intraneural) the main peripheral nerve or its branches in:

1. Hansen's neuritis.
2. Post-traumatic perinural adhesions or adhesive neuritis.
3. Painful neuromas.
4. Non-specific peripheral neuritis.
5. Meralgia paresthetica.
6. Radiculitis—mostly following degenerative rupture of disc or altered joint conditions.
7. Entrapment neuropathy.

RESISTANT (NON-SPECIFIC OR AT TIMES SPECIFIC) BACKACHE

Resistant specific or at times non-specific backache, a truly unsolved problem, does respond to infiltration of corticoid (mostly without any true explanation). It may be given as local infiltration at the most tender spot, into the tendor and/or triggering nodule, or as epidural injections (also see the chapter on "Spine").

SKIN CONDITIONS

Local corticoid infilteration has been reported to have a definite role in certain skin conditions:

1. Disseminated lupus erythematosus
2. Eczematous conditions
3. Keloid
4. Non-specific dermatitis
5. Leucoderma
6. Hard and soft corn
7. Alopecia

OPHTHALMIC CONDITION

Corticoid infiltration has been used in corneal ulcer to prevent scar. For the same purpose it has also been used in post-operative or post-traumatic ophthalmic conditions.

GYNAECOLOGICAL CONDITIONS

A cocktail consisting of hydrocortisone acetate 1 cc and water for injection 9 cc plus crystalline penicillin/streptomycin plus hyaluronidase has been used earlier for hydrotubation in cases of tubal blockage, which has been replaced nowadays by instillation of placentrex. Hydrocortisone acetate, sometimes, is given after tubal microsurgery.

It has been given intrafoetally in cases of post-maturity due to anencephaly.

REFLEX SYMPATHETIC DYSTROPHY SYNDROME (RSDS)

In managing early stage of post-traumatic RSDS regional intravenous blocks of a mixture of corticoids and lidocaine have been found to be highly effective. It is recommended as the first choice treatment because it is simple, safe and well tolerated (Tountas et al 1993).

TRIAL INDICATIONS

For the conditions where no specific explanation for the pain and/or stiffness around the joint or bursa, tendon or ligaments, muscle, bone or subcutaneous tissue is available, a trial local infiltration of corticoid cocktail in and around the affected area is recommended. In such circumstances usually one to two injections should be tried. Depending upon the response further injections may be given.

In osteochondrosis of scaphoid (Preiser's disease), lunate (Kienbock's disease) and navicular (Kohler's disease), trial injections of corticoid must be given before embarking on surgery.

In ischio-gluteal bursitis (weaver's bottom) and epiphysitis of metatarsal (Freiberg's infarction) cocktail infiltration may give relief. Similarly, in painful hallux valgus, hallux rigidus, tailor's bunion (in varus angulation of the fifth toe) and inter-digital neuroma (Morton's toe) there may be trial indications of corticoid cocktail.

Injections of corticoids can also provide relief but has been occasionally objected for its effect in causing atrophy of fat and leaving small depigmented patches in the skin. In various bursitis like olecranon bursitis (student's elbow), prepatellar bursitis (housemaid's knee) and other bursitis around the knee joint, aspiration followed by intrabursal injection of corticoid cocktail may by effective.

In spastic flat foot, if the spasm is dominating, infiltration of lignocain into the sinus tarsi gives immediate relief. In such cases infiltration of long acting local anaesthetic may provide lasting results.

CHAPTER 5

Contraindications for Local Corticosteroid Therapy

GENERAL INFECTIONS

It is an absolute contraindication to all corticosteroid therapy.

- **Localized infective focus** (mainly pyogenic) even at a distance from the joint to be infiltrated (*e.g.* skin, ENT, urinary, pulmonary).

- Any haemostatic disorder: If the patient is under anticoagulants, there is possibility of developing haemarthrosis. Further, since blood is an excellent culture medium, there is risk of quick proliferation of infective organisms, hence it is a relative contraindication to local corticoid therapy because of the risk of infection.

- Diabetes: One must be cautious in diabetic patients. Even when controlled, it can favour post-infiltrative infections. Repeated infiltrations can cause diabetic disequilibrium.

- Prosthetic replacements: All periprosthetic corticosteriod therapy should be abandoned.

- Inflammatory processes associated with metabolic disorders, collagen diseases, osteoarthritis and similar conditions may be an indication in carefully selected cases, otherwise it is contraindication. The depth and extent of inflammation and circulatory changes can be assessed by some non-invasive investigative technique, *e.g.* thermography.

- Severe joint disruption.

- Uncorrected static deformity.

- Severe osteoporosis of bones adjacent to joints.

- Unstable joints.

- Neuropathic joints.

- Traumatic arthritis due to intra-articular fractures.

CHAPTER 6

Intra-articular Hyaluronic Acid

In the last decade the role of hyaluronic acid in the management of osteoarthritis and rheumatoid arthritis has been much emphasised.

Hylans is the generic name of hyaluronate. Hyaluronate is a glucosaminoglycan with a repeating disaccharide structure that is composed of D-glucuronic acid in linkage to N-acetyl-D-glucosamine. Free hyaluronic acid occurs only in laboratory conditions, hence hyaluronate or hyaluronan are recommended terms. Combining 12,500 disaccharide units produces one molecule of hyaluronan with a molecular weight of about 5 million. Hyaluronate is a hydrophilic polysaccharide belonging to the group of glucosaminoglycans. When hydrated it assumes a larger molecular volume, and thus occupies a large spheroidial domain. The molecular network of hyaluronate is permeable to the molecules which are smaller than the network elements. This network works as a sieve for larger molecules.

The hyaluronan solution possesses both elastic and viscous properties. This elastoviscosity of hyaluronan varies according to motion and shear forces. In presence of slower motion and lower shear forces, the solution behaves like a viscous fluid (which denotes that the mechanical energy is dissipated as heat through the movement of the network). whereas with more rapid motion and higher shear forces, its behaviour resembles the features of an elastic body (which means that the mechanical energy is stored in the molecular network). Thus, diluted solutions of hyaluronan of sufficient molecular weight can function as effective lubricant when movements are slow and as shock absorbers when movements are fast.

Synovial fluid permeates the superficial layer of the articular cartilage as well as the intracellular matrix of the synovial tissue and capsule. This effectively fills the collagen matrix of the intracellular space with viscoelastic hyaluronan. The joint movements generate a flow of synovial fluid maintaining a continuous exchange of hyaluronan between the synovial fluid and the intercellular fluid of the joint tissue.

The molecular mass of hyaluronan in a normal joint is about 4 to 5 million. The theological properties of arthritic synovial fluid are less than that of normal fluid, hence a substance intended for viscosupplementation must have considerably greater elastoviscosity than the synovial fluid present in an arthritic joint. This was achieved by the development of a highly elastoviscous solution composed of two crosslinked hyaluronans.

VISCOSUPPLEMENTATION

The concept of viscosupplementation for the joint was developed by Endre A. Balazs and his co-workers in 1960s.

Hylan is an easily deformable gel with fluid like properties. In 1960s the development of hyaluronan, derived from human umblical cord and rooster combs, for medical use was begun (Biotrics, Inc., Arlington M.A).

Hyaluronate is present in synovial fluid as the major macromolecular component and is responsible for the intrinsic viscoelasticity.

Because of its hyaluronic acid content, joint fluid acts as a viscous lubricant during slow movement of the joint, as in walking, and as an elastic shock absorber during rapid movement, as in running. It is considered not only a joint lubricant, but also a physiological factor in the trophic status of cartilage. Hyaluronic acid has a very high water binding capacity. When 1 g of hyaluronic acid is dissolved in physiological saline, it occupies three litres of solution. The estimated total hyaluronic acid in a human knee joint is 4 to 8 mg (Adams et al 1995).

Decrease in concentration of hyaluronate is more important factor in the arthropathies than the observed reduction in molecular weight (Balazs EA 1974).

MECHANISM OF ANALGESIC ACTION OF HYLAN

The exact mechanism of analgesic action of hylan is not known. It is assumed that it acts by virtue of restoring joint homeostasis, which leads to decrease in pain.

The joint motion creates an exertive force, which drives fluid out of joint.

The most significant force, which drives fluid out of a joint is the pressure exerted during joint motion. Lymph channels drain out the fluid in the joint, by which homeostasis is maintained. When the fluid accumulates in joint due to any pathology, the concentration of hyaluronic acid decreases, which leads to a vicious circle. In arthralgia due to pain and increase in fluid volume, the joint movements decrease. In such situation the injected hylan restores the theological properties of synovial fluid and thus may improve the fluid mechanics in the joint, which in turn may improve the joint movements and reduce the pain.

Probably, the ability of hylan to restore joint homeostasis is responsible for its analgesic effects, however, as shown experimentally in rats (Pozo et al 1997) it also has a direct analgesic effect on joint nociceptors.

ROLE OF HYALURONIC ACID IN OSTEOARTHRITIS

Hyaluronic acid (HA), one of the most important components of synovial fluid, is usually accepted as the protector of articular cartilage and soft tissue surfaces from injury during joint function. HA is an important, although minor component of the articular cartilage matrix, and it plays an important role in the aggregation of proteoglycans (Balazs et al 1966) suggested that a 1-2 μ thick layer, which adheres to the articular cartilage surface, may contain HA, which may protect cartilage from wear and may also act as a shock absorber, protecting the cartilage from shock thrusts. Disturbances in the HA level in the synovial fluid may result in damage to the surface layer, and due to changes in the permeability proteins and other HMW (High Molecular Weight) substances may permeate into the cartilage matrix. Therefore, injection of HMW—HA may restore the damaged HA layer on the surface of articular cartilage, alleviating the arthritic condition and retarding the progress of the disease.

The overall role of the elastoviscous fluid, injected into the knee joint, has been deduced as to supplement and restore, the lubricating, protecting and shock absorbing properties of synovial fluid, which are compromised in osteoarthritis. After biomatrix scientists introduced this system (in clinical medicine) known as viscosupplimentation, it has been variously observed in relieving the pain and improving the mobility in osteoarthritic joint.

In the beginning HA was extracted from bovine vitreous humor (had a MW of 15-20 $\times$ 10^4 and a protein content of approximately 10%), later Balazs et al (1972) purified HA from human umblical cord and rooster combs with a high MW (100-300 $\times$ 10^4), high viscosity and protein content of less than 1%, and named them HA, Healone. After obtaining good results with injecting the HA into arthritic and/or traumatic joint in the animals, intra-articular injection of HA was also observed to be effective in human being (Helfet 1974). At least there was no aggrevation of the symptoms after HA injection.

In most of the cases the effects of HA injection was seen in two days, however the effects lasted variably from one week to 12 months (on an average 8 weeks).

CORTICOIDS VS HYALURONIC ACID

Like the effect of corticoids many patients begin to respond only after few HA injections but few may require even 8-10 injections to show the effect. However, the long-term effect may be satisfactory, especially in osteoarthritis. In animal (rabbits) repeated HA intra-articular injection was found to have a preventive effect (Namiki et al 1975).

Side Effects

Experimentally, even twice a week HA intra-articular injection for 6 months have been tolerated well in dogs without any side effect, however, in human beings 16 HA injections did not produce any adverse effects.

Intra-articular HA did not prove effective in osteo-arthritic joints with effusion, probably because the scheduled effect of HA is nullified by the excessive joint fluid.

The efficacy and long-term benefit of intra-articular hyaluronic acid injection have not been yet clearly established. Further, the disadvantages of this treatment include the need for a minimum of initial three injections. Unlike corticoids, HA disappears from the joint cavity within a few days of intra-articular injection, hence long lasting effect of HA cannot be explained by direct action of HA alone. Probably, it normalizes synovial fluid production and helps in the reconstruction of barrier protecting the synovial membrane and cartilage surface.

As corticoids do, HA does not have anti-inflammatory effects. Hence, if cocktail of HA and corticoids is injected, the overall results becomes superior than of either alone. Further the dose of corticoids is reduced (half or even less) in future requirements to have some effect, thereby the possible adverse side-effects of repeated corticoids injection can be avoided.

If compared for effects in osteo-arthritic knee there is hardly any difference between patients treated with intra-articular injections of Hylan G-F$_{20}$ (one course of three weekly injections) and those treated with corticosteroid (two to three weekly injection) with respect to pain relief or functional improvement by 6 to 9 months follow-up.

A comparative experimental study with histopathologic evaluations have been shown that corticoid is effective in the treatment of cartilage degeneration and inflammation early in the course of septic arthritis, whereas the therapeutic effect of hyaluronon is higher late in the course of the disease. However, further multicornered studies are required to draw proper conclusion (Karak et al 2001).

As a practical approach it appears that for a knee with effusion, corticosteroids injection should be considered and for symptomatic dry knee hyaluronic acid injection may be more favourable choice.

21

CHAPTER 7

Methodology

PREPARATION

The part to be injected must be assessed thoroughly prior to injection, keeping in view:

1. Condition of skin at and around the point of prick.
2. Presence of infective disease in the joint or the enviornment (which is a contraindication).
3. Point of maximum tenderness (where relative and trial indications are laid down) which should be marked either with skin marker pencil or by nail edge (which does not disappear while preparing the skin for injection).
4. Accessibility of the joint i.e. preferable route of infiltration. The part must be fully exposed (as far as practicable as if preparing for the orthopaedic operation in that area).

EQUIPMENTS

- A sterile split towel.
- Two syringes, the pistons of which move smoothly.
- A 20-gauge needle is most commonly used, although needle from 19 to 24 gauge may sometimes be required.

POSITION OF THE PATIENT

Many a times it becomes difficult to negotiate a needle through a joint space only for the faulty position of the patient. Hence, it is imperative that patient should be placed in a position which allows easy approach to the joint concerned (vide individual joint).

SOAP WATER CLEANING OF THE PART

This easy and always available procedure must be taken as mandatory. The fat solvent effect of the soap cleans the skin creases much more effectively, comparable to or even more than any other detergent or anti septic solution. Areas well above and well below the site of prick should be thoroughly scrubbed, cleaned and washed out. Hair must be shaved from hairy areas.

CERTAIN CONSIDERATIONS IN RELATION TO INTRA-ARTICULAR AND ALLIED INJECTIONS

1. Corticosteroid injections must be given in an operation theatre environment in an aseptic surrounding.

   There is all danger of introducing infection through local injection therapy, **NOT** only the millions of tiny microcrystals of corticosteroids physically protect the infective organisms from the access of the body defences, but the corticosteroids themselves suppress the local immune inflammatory response to infection. Hence, strict aseptic technique is mandatory.

2. The syringe, needle and other equipments must be thoroughly sterilized by autoclaving or prolonged boiling for minimum of 30 minutes or sterilised double layered packed disposable equipments should be used.

3. The joint along with wide areas in the surroundings must be thoroughly cleaned by repeated soapwater/detergents and/or chlorhexidine gluconate-cetrimide and rectified spirit (available as savlon) and/or microbicidal solutions (e.g. povidone-iodine available as Betadine) or allied antiseptics.

4. The stopper of corticosteroid/methyl prednisolone acetate or hydrocortisone acetate and local anaesthetics vials must be thoroughly cleaned by above lotions.

5. The surgeon must scrub thoroughly and use a pair of sterilised gloves.

6. After antiseptic procedures, as far as possible, always avoid touching the part to be injected. However, if it is essential to localise the point of prick, an antiseptic swab mopping must precede the needle prick.

7. It is beneficial to use a sharp, fine needle (20 to 24 gauges). Though hydrocortisone acetate is a suspension, we had not a single occasion to repent for not using the wide-bore needle for intra-articular injection. The prick remains almost painless.

   Thoroughly sterilised double-layered packed disposable syringes, needles and gloves should be used.

8. A controlled sharp quick push through the joint space gives very little trouble to the patient. Whatever possible, the joint fluid should be aspirated, inspected and sent for culture. If the fluid is opaeque or other than the normal synovial fluid look, corticoid should not be injected, rather inject some antibiotics if there is any doubt of any infection (e.g. kanamycin).

9. Always avoid touching the bone or cartilage surface by the needle-end. Somehow or other, it hurts the patient instantaneously and pain persists for varying periods, sometimes even days together. In certain cases effusion and swelling develop. Of course, it settles with assurances, ice-cold compress, rest to the part and analgesic. Theoretical risks always exist causing damage to articular cartilage by the sharp needle point and also by the chemical activity of the corticosteroids which is likely to soften the articular cartilage predisposing to tear.

10. Local anaesthetic is not necessary if proper techniques are applied. However, when it is essential, keep the needle in situ after injecting local anaesthetic, detach the syringe to load the corticoid or cocktail; do not leave the end of the needle open to exterior; rather, put a sterilized small cotton wool over the needle-end to avoid contamination with the environmental air.

    One dilemma in using the local anaesthetic may disappoint the patient against which they should be warned. With local anaesthetics the patient may feel instant relief, but pain returns after the anaesthetics effect wears off.

11. It has been seen that in an over-enthusiastic attempt to inject the last droplet of drug, some air is pushed into. It must be avoided, at least it is going to increase the bulk in the joint space besides potentially carrying the possibility of infection (unless it is done in the modern operation theatre enviornment).

12. Aftet taking out the needle, few droplets/drops of blood may come out. A gentle, local to and fro massage automatically seals the passage. However, it is always better to seal the prick with tincture of benzoin or povidine-iodine.

    Be cautious where you are injecting in the joint where someone else has previously given an injection and when the technique might not have been that meticulous as should be. In such cases send the adequate fluid for culture.

13. Following injection of corticoid ask the patient to gently move the joint or part as far as practicable. This helps in dispersal of the injected material. If needed the joint should be moved few times passively.

14. Patient must not be allowed to be up and about immediately after the prick. There can be psychological fear, vasovagal attack and allergic reactions to lidocaine hydrochloride or other materials used.

15. The patient should be restrained from immediate vigorous use of the limb or exercises. About 24 hours abstinence from vigorous activities or exercises provides comfort to the patient in subsequent activities or physiotherapy. This helps by providing a time for biological adaptation. In any case the patient should be firmly warned not to apply untoward stress on the joint injected.

16. More than one joint can be injected at a time but let it be not more than four joints in one sitting e.g. in rheumatoid arthritis. After all we are dealing with living human creatures and the patient may not be able to use his several joints for variable period. As such even 125 mg of hydrocortisone acetate or more (and comparable amount of the corticoids) can be used at a time without any complication.

17. If there is pain after intra-articular injections, initially ice pack application helps in allaying pain. After 12 to 16 hours, hot moist fomentation may be useful. It helps in allaying the associated inflammatory process, if any. Further, counter-irritant effect of heat allays the pain following the prick.

18. There is hardly any systemic effect of local corticoid injection, however, rarely improvements occur in other (than one injected) joints, which may be due to the systemic effects of the injected corticoids ultimately entering the blood stream with the same explanation. There may be very rare risk of adrenal cortical suppression after repeated corticoid injections, and it may produce theoretical hazards of inadequate adrenal cortical response to the stresses.

19. One should always be apprehensive of aggravating the infection after injecting into an already infected joint. However, sometimes the patients of chronic arthritis with damaged joints (e.g. rheumatoid arthritis) already treated by oral corticoids do not manifest the systemic constitutional features of infection, and in such cases it is difficult to clinically diagnose the pyogenic infection of the joint, and one may inject the corticoids in such infected joints. However, it is always safe to aspirate the fluid and send for culture before injection therapy.

    Sometimes after local injection, the pain increases with features of inflammation, giving rise to worries about iatrogenic infection. However, microcrystalline suspensions of corticoids may induce temporary crystal synovitis like gout producing the inflammatory features. This should be managed by rest, NSAID, cold compress, and reassurance along with prophylactic antibiotics.

20. Like compuMed (computer controlled local anaesthetic delivery system—a revolution, any system that allows to easily deliver virtually painfree injections of local anaesthetic) corticoid can also be given which will have much patient's acceptability. The compuMed system provides microprocessor control for more precise and predictable drug delivery.

SITES FOR INJECTION

In orthopaedic practice, corticoids have been used for:

- Intra-articular
- Peri-articular
- Intra-tendinous (?) – very cautiously since it may predipose to rupture of the tendon.
- Peri-tendinous
- Intra-nodular
- Perinodular injection
- Intraneural—e.g. in Hansen's neuritis into peripheral nerves (e.g. ulnar, lateral popliteal nerves, etc)
- Perineural—epidural injection

In most of the joints, intra-articular injections are needed, but few joints suffering from peri-articular adhesive capsulitis lesions (e.g. shoulder joint) do require peri-articular infiltration. In selecting the site of injection for a joint following points must be considered: -

i. Approach should be direct into the joint.

ii. Prick must avoid major blood vessels and nerves.

iii. As far as possible, joint-line should be first located.

If blood uniformly mixed with joint fluid is aspirated, suspect trauma (haemarthrosis—blood appears more thicker and veinous and with sparkling fat globules) or bleeding disease. In such situation haemarthrosis should be aspirated, and some prophylactic antibiotic may be injected but corticoids should not be injected.

Possibility of damage to articular cartilage by the sharp point of needle always exists, which must be avoided as far as possible. It is liable to predispose softening of the cartilage (further accentuated by the chemical activities of the injected corticoids).

After corticoid injection there is the possibility of aspetic necrosis of the joint surface due to infarction of the subchondral bone. However, such lesions may exist prior to injection as well e.g. in hips, knees, ankles especially in severe rheumatoid arthritis, and cartilage breakdown after local corticoid injection in these joints may be just coincidental.

Sometimes following the injections of long acting corticosteroids in superficial joints (e.g. knee, PIP or DIP joints) some of the injected material may leak out through the injection tract and cause some discoloration (e.g. whitish patch) and atrophy of overlying skin with increased transparancy.

CHAPTER 8

Shoulder Joint

In all approaches the point of prick should be ascertained and marked by skin pencil or nail edge before preparing the part antiseptically.

Anterior Approach

The patient lies supine with arm by the side of chest and shoulder girdle well supported on the sand bag. Feel the tip of the coracoid process, just outside it, a narrow depression can be felt, extending more downwards than upwards. The fingertip can be hardly insinuated in it. Mark it by skin pencil or nail edge before preparing it antiseptically. In the depression, the needle should be pushed posteriorly with slight outward and downward inclination. Usually no resistance is felt and needle may be pushed upto hilt (Figure 8.1).

Posterior Approach

This approach is suitable for periarthritic infiltration. However, it can also be used for injecting into the joint. Patient lies by the side with the joint to be injected above. Posterior

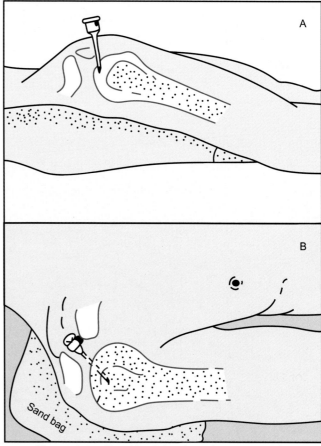

Figure 8.1: Shoulder joint (anterior approach). Viewed from side (A); from above (B)

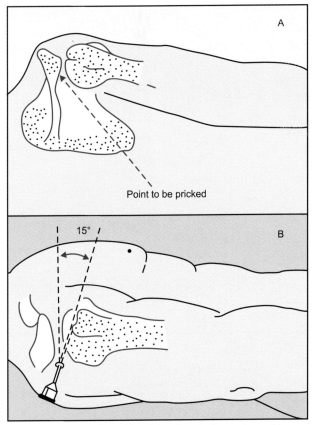

Figure 8.2: Shoulder joint (posterior approach). Viewed from back (A); from above (B)

acromion angle is felt. Just lateral to and behind it, a finger-tip can be insinuated into a depression. Mark it before preparing for injection. A needle may be introduced through it, anteriorly with very little (about 15°) downward inclination (Figure 8.2).

PERI-ARTHRITIC INFILTRATION

The patient lies on his side with the arm to be injected resting on the side of chest. Posterior acromion angle is felt. Just lateral and behind it, finger-tip can be insinuated into a depression. Through it, a needle is pushed anteriorly with 15 to 20 degrees downwards and outwards inclination (Figure 8.3). Pricking up to the hilt of the needle is without any resistance. As the drug is injected one can see slight puffing just anteriorly. This is due to pouching out of sub-acromion bursa.

Peri-arthritic infiltration may be done in sitting posture also, however, lying down position should be preferred. Patient sits on a stool against the back of the upright of a chair, kept infront of him. The lower portion of both forearms rest on the arms of the chair from behind. Automatically, the

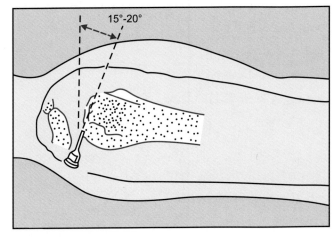

Figure 8.3: Shoulder joint—approach for periarthritic infiltration

arms lie in slight flexion, abduction and internal rotation position.

Feel the posterior angle of acromion. Just below and outside it, a sharp depression is felt. Push the needle forward with a slight medial and downward inclination (Figure 8.4).

Antero-lateral Approach

In bicipital tenosynovitis, corticoid infiltration can be done into the sheath of biceps tendon as well as in bicipital groove. The patient lies supine with a sandbag beneath the shoulder. The most tendor point is sought on the anterolateral slope of the shoulder top. Occasionally a thickened, tender band can be rolled under the finger (Figure 8.4).

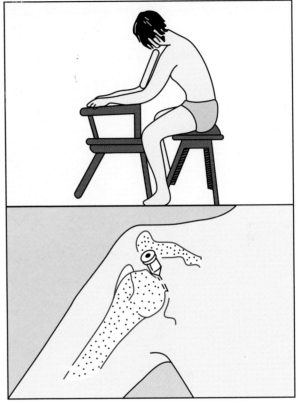

Figure 8.4: Shoulder joint—approach in sitting position

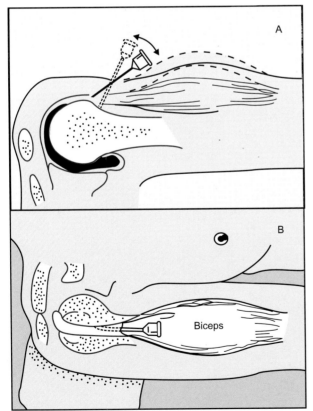

Figure 8.5: Infiltration for bicipital tenosynovitis. Viewed from side (A); from above (B)

The needle should be pushed from below upwards with an inclination backwards and laterally for infiltration into the sheath (Figure 8.5). As the sheath is entered into, one can see and test, to and fro movements of the detached needle with contraction and relaxation of biceps tendon. After injecting into the sheath the needle can be pushed further backwards to enter into the bicipital groove, a bony resistance is felt as the floor of bicipital groove is reached. The tendon should not be infiltrated into, only it should be bathed from all around.

Intra-articular distention in the management of capsulitis of the shoulder (6 ml 0.25% bupivacaine and 3 ml of air) has been found to be superior to the intra-articular injection of steroid alone (40 mgm triamcinolone acetonide in 1 ml). However, more improvement was observed when steroid and distension were combined, with distension probably acting synergistically (Jacobs L G H et al 1991). Posterior route to gleno-humeral joint should be employed for injection and distension.

CHAPTER 9

Elbow Joint

Elbow is a composite joint having ulno-humeral, radio-humeral and radio-ulnar components. These have continuous and communicating synovial reflections. Therefore, if the drug is injected into one component, it easily spreads into other compartments, unless there is intra-articular adhesions.

Lateral Approach

Lateral approach is through radio-humeral compartment. The patient lies supine. The arm is kept in slight internal rotation at shoulder. The elbow is flexed 30 to 40 degree from zero extension, with forearm is midprone position. A transverse slit can be felt at the posterolateral aspect just below the lateral epicondylar region. Further confirmation can be done by rotating the forearm in which radial head is felt rotating just beneath the slit. The needle is pushed into the slit having a direction anteriorly with about 20 degree upward inclination (Figure 9.1).

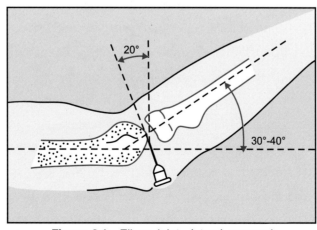

Figure 9.1: Elbow joint—lateral approach

Posterior Approach

The patient lies on the side with the affected limb above. Elbow is flexed about 45 degree with forearm in midprone position. The olecranon tip stands prominent. On either side of the olecranon process a vertical slit can be felt. At a convenient point along the slit, a needle can be pushed on either side of the olecranon, having a direction downwards and towards mid-line (Figure 9.2).

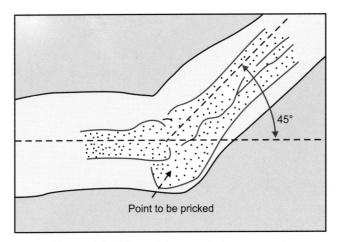

Figure 9.2: Elbow joint—posterior approach

Lateral Epicondylitis (Extra-articular Tennis Elbow)

Lateral epicondylitis (tennis elbow) has been recogonized for over 100 years. It is an enthesopathy of the common extensors origin in the lateral epicondylar region, however, its pathogenesis is not clear. It has been also recognized as an overuse syndrome (repetitive stress disorder) due to repetitive tension overloading of the wrist extensor origin at the lateral epicondylar region.

First clinical description of lateral epicondylitis was given by Runge in 1873. More than 40 different types of treatment have been used alone or in combinations e.g. anti-inflammatory drugs, steroids, physiotherapy techniques, cast immobilisation, orthosis, surgery, and less conventional methods such as radiotherapy, acupuncture and vitamins (Labelle et al 1992). Recently extracorporeal shock-wave therapy (ESWT) has been used in tennis elbow. The mobile lithotriper (2000 shock waves at 2.5 bars of air pressure with a frequency of 8-10 Hz—a total of three sittings at an interval of 2 weeks, each lasting for three to four minutes is an effective way of treating tennis elbow and plantar fascitis but it requires, further trials for authentication. However, it is much costly as compared to corticosteroids injection (100 times) and also less effective. By and large injection of corticosteroids alongwith hyaluronidase and local anaesthetic is more effective treatment of tennis elbow.

In the elbow region, it is the commonest indication. Infiltration in such cases is done in and around the origin of common extensors from anteroinferior aspect of lateral epicondylar region. The patient

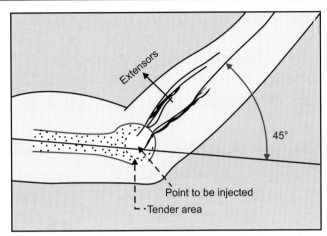

Figure 9.3: Elbow joint—approach of extra-articular tennis elbow

lies supine. The elbow is kept in 45 degrees flexion in midprone position. The antero-inferior part of lateral epicondylar region is easily felt. Palpate over the bony region and its adjoining area for locating the maximum tenderness. The most tendor point is directly injected pushing the needle almost upto subperiosteal region. The adjoining areas should also be infiltrated (Figure 9.3). It is better to manipulate at the elbow in the same sitting. Hold the hand of the patient in your right hand in the handshake position. Support the elbow from behind by your left hand. While gently rotating the forearm and flexing/extending at elbow, give a sudden jerky extension to the elbow. You may hear a mild click. Quite often it gives good relief, probably by viture of breaking the fibrotic adhesions.

Olecranon Bursitis

Olecranon bursitis is the inflammation of the bursa overlying the olecranon process caused by repetitive or even acute trauma. It presents as a more or less round tense, fluctuant (may not be demonstrable), tender swelling. It should be aspirated from the nondependent side (to avoid leakage after withdrawing the needle). Usually no local anaesthetic is required. The aspiration needle is advanced while maintaining negative pressure in the syringe. When the fluid starts flowing, the needle is no longer advanced further. If the fluid is clear, the needle should be left in situ and other syringe containing the steroid is changed to inject it slowly after the aspirate stopped flowing. It may prevent recurrence. If the fluid is not clear it should be sent for examination and culture.

Medial Epicondylitis (Golfer's elbow, Pitcher's elbow,
Little League elbow syndrome)

It is an overuse syndrome, common in young persons and is caused by chronic tension stress injuries, repetitive tension overloading of the flexor-pronator muscles at or near its origin from the medial epicondyle.

When the problem does not improve with non-invasive methods (as noted in lateral epicondylitis) local infiltration of the corticoid cocktail should be done in the flexor-pronator muscles origin complex just at and near the medial epicondyle.

Method

Patient lies supine with shoulder abducted (by 90°), elbow flexed by 40° 'and forearm supinated. The medial epicondyle is palpated and maximum tendor point is spotted and marked by skin pencil or nail edge. After preparing the skin antiseptically the needle is pushed from just below the medial epicondylar tip in the upward and anterior direction. Just before reaching the bone the medicine is pushed infiltrating the zone.

CHAPTER 10

Wrist Joint

For all practical purposes, wrist joint behaves as a composite joint, consisting of radio-carpal joint, inter-carpal joints and inferior radio-ulnar joint. These have inter-communicating synovial reflections. But, inter-carpal joints being very snugly spaced, drugs pushed into these joints can hardly reach the inferior radio-ulnar joint. In most of the cases requiring corticoid injection, the inferior radio-ulnar joint is at fault, especially after trauma in and around the wrist joint.

APPROACHES

In post traumatic conditions (of which the most common is malunited Colles fracture) pressure at the tip of the ulnar styloid process initiates pain and is most tendor. It is either due to fibrous healing of the avulsed ulnar styloid process, or mild persistent subluxation of inferior radio-ulnar joint, or inferior radio-ulnar traumatic synovitis or arthritis. In such conditions local infiltration beneath and around the tip of ulnar styloid process can be done directly. For injecting into the wrist joint and/ or into the inferior radio-ulnar joint following methods may be followed.

a. The patient lies supine and keeps the wrist in prone position. Feel the ulnar styloid process. Just beneath and behind it there is a depression. Through it push the needle radialwards with about 20 degree of upward and foreward inclination (Figure 10.1).

b. In fully prone position of the hand, wrist is flexed to about 20 to 30 degree. About 0.5 cm below the mid-interstyloid line an yield or depression can be felt on the dorsum of wrist. The needle can be pushed through the gap almost anteriorly with 15 degree upward inclination (Figure 10.2).

de-QUERVAIN'S DISEASE

In the wrist region, perhaps, the most common use of corticoid injection is in the de-Quervain's

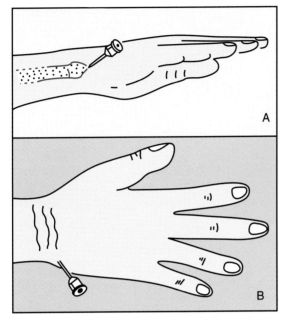

Figure 10.1: Wrist joint—approach from ulnar side. Lateral view (A); dorsal view (B)

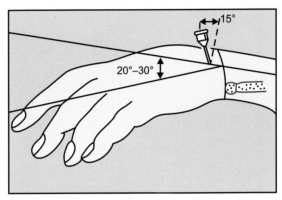

Figure 10.2: Wrist joint—approach from dorsum

disease (stenosing tenosynovitis of the abductor pollicis longus and extensor pollicis brevis tendon) and ganglion. The firm and tendor swelling in this disease is obvious above the radial styloid process (Figure 10.3).

Method

The patient lies supine. In mid-prone position of the hand, the needle is pushed, starting about 1cm above the styloid process, below upwards in the direction of abductor pollicis longus tendon. When the sheath is supposed to be entered into, the needle should be disconnected from the syringe and the patient is asked to abduct the extent the thumb repeatedly. With each movement the needle moves to and fro with playing of the tendon. This must be tested before injecting the drug.

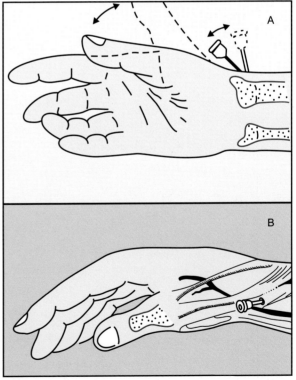

Figure 10.3: Approach for de-Quervain's disease. Viewed from side (A); needle into tendon sheath (B)

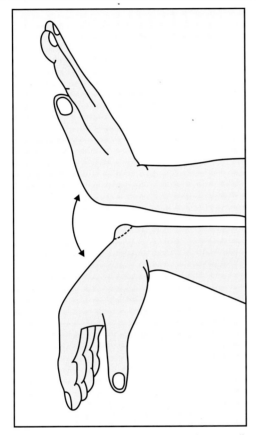

Figure 10.4: Test showing intra-articular ganglion

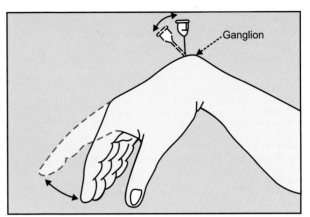

Figure 10.5: Injection into ganglion of extensor tendon of index finger

Another common indication around the wrist is for a ganglion, (Figures 10.4 and 5). Ganglion must be pithed and injected into directly. For the ganglion associated with any tendon, to and fro movements of the needle after penetrating the sheath of that tendon should be tested with the movement of that particular tendon. The ganglion should be made prominent by contracting the particular tendon before injecting into it. If it lies deep to the tendon, it will not become prominent, but will be fixed with contraction of the tendon; which will facilitate the injection. Ganglion communicating with the wrist or carpal joints diminish in size or disappear following dorsiflexion of the wrist joint. Hence, it should be made prominent by palmar-flexing the wrist before injection.

By the use of hyaluronidase the results of ganglion aspiration can be improved. The good effect has also been observed in de-Quervain's disease.

METACARPOPHALANGEAL JOINTS AND INTER-PHALANGEAL JOINTS

Flexing the particular joint by about 45 degree, a narrow transverse slit can be felt by gentle palpation, especially by the nail edge. Confirm it by repeatedly flexing and extending the joint. The fine needle can be pushed into the joint through the slit. Periarticular infiltration should also be done, if there is suspicion of particular adhesions (Figure 10.6).

The metacarpophalangeal and inter-phalangeal joints can also be approached through the slit, felt on either side of joint, in about 45 degree flexed position of that particular joint (Figure 10.7).

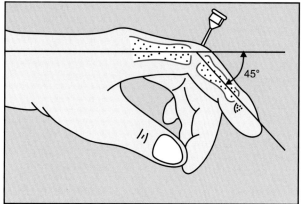

Figure 10.6: Approach to inter-phalangeal joint from dorsum

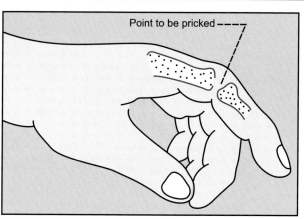

Figure 10.7: Approach to inter-phalangeal joint from side

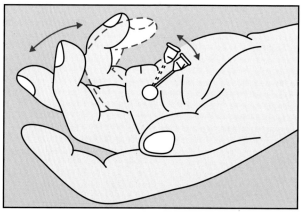

Figure 10.8: Approach for trigger ring finger

Trigger Thumb/Finger (Figure 10.8)

A common indication of corticoid injection in thumb or finger is trigger-thumb and trigger-finger. In this condition the patient complains of temporary locking of the thumb or finger in the flexed position, to a varying extent. The finger can be extended by using more power for extension and jerky release is felt. One can palpate the firm tender nodule in the course of the concerned tendon, usually at the root of thumb on the pulmar aspect, and along the lines of ring and middle fingers, distal to the distal palmar crease. These nodules are due to localized circumferential fibrosis in the tendon-sheath. Usually, injection is most effective within 3 to 4 weeks of the onset of pain and early triggering of the finger. As the nodule gets firmer, infiltrating of corticoids may be effective in reducing the pain to varying extent, but nodule persists and pain usually recurs. In such cases surgical slitting-open of the tendon-sheath in the nodular region gives almost cure.

Method

By a direct approach just proximal or distal to the nodule, the local anaesthetic may be infiltrated by the needle. The nodule is pithed and the tendon-sheath is entered into. A to and fro movements of needle is tested with excursion of that particular tendon before injecting the drug (Figure 10.8).

CHAPTER 11

Hip Joint

The degenerative changes in the hip joints, either primary or secondary to various conditions, are quite common. The corticoid injection is effective in degenerative arthrosis of the hip joint too. However, because of the difficult access to the hip-joint proper, specially in non-distended capsule, intra-articular injection of corticoids could not be that popular. The approaches for injecting into the hip joint can be anterior or posterolateral.

Anterior Approach (Figure 11.1)

The patient lies supine. Feel the femoral pulsation just below and outside the mid-inguinal point. About a finger-breadth out to it, will be the suitable point to approach the hip joint i.e. about 2 to 3 cm below the anterior superior iliac spine and 2 to 3 cm lateral to the femoral pulse. Push the needle posteriorly with an inclination downwards and medially at an angle of about 60 degree with the skin through the hip capsule until bone is reached. Then the tip of needle is slightly withdrawn. In lucky situation, a drop or

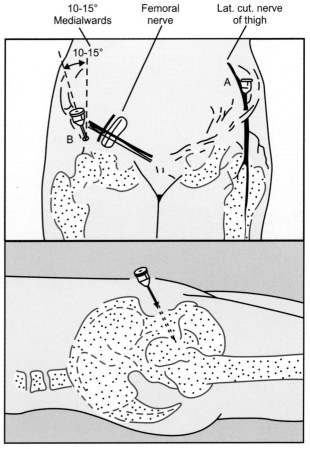

Figure 11.1: Above (right side)—anterior approach to hip joint; (left side)—approach for meralgia paresthetica. Below—anterior approach to hip joint: viewed from side

two of synovial fluid can be aspirated, which will confirm the penetration into the joint capsule. Under image intensifier, however, the needle can be manipulated comparatively easily into the hip joint. Even if bigger dose of corticoid is injected, the ball and socket joint of such a big dimension perhaps hurdles in spreading the drug over the inflamed synovial reflections of the joint.

Lateral Approach (Figure 11.2)

It is also a difficult approach, however with a slender long needle, hip can be penetrated into. In this approach there is advantage that the needle follow the bone to the hip joint. The patient lies in lateral position with the joint to be injected kept above. The needle is inserted just anterior to the greater trochanter in a sagittal direction pointing towards the mid-inguinal point. The needle tip slides anterior to the periosteum of the femoral neck and enters the hip joint space anteriorly.

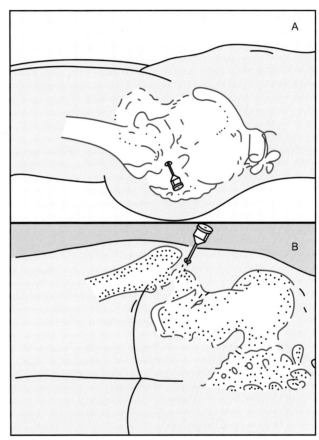

Figure 11.2: Postero-lateral approach. Viewed from above (A); from back (B)

The corticoid injection is also given for meralgia paresthetica (entrapment of lateral cutaneous nerve of thigh under the outer end of inguinal ligament). The injection should be in cocktail of corticoid, hyaluronidase and lignocaine. The injection may be effective when given in early stage. Later on surgery seems to be inevitable, even though the result may not be uniformly good.

Method (Figure 11.1)

The patient lies supine. Select a point about a finger breadth medial to anterior iliac spine. Push the needle at this point with an inclination down to about subcutaneous depth. Slowly infiltrate corticoid cocktail vertically downwards in the area of about 3 cm at the depth of about 1 cm.

CHAPTER 12

Knee Joint

Perhaps no other joint has been more popular a place for intra-articular injection than the knee joint, causes being:

1. The joint line is most easily felt and approachable and the joint spaces can be easily delineated percutaneously.
2. The knee joint is the most common site for degenerative changes especially in the subjects with Asian culture. In these countries, social and religious obligations demand, quite often, squatting and sitting in **Budha's position** (crossed-legged position), which are definitely strenuous to the joints.
3. The articular surfaces being mostly flat, the injected drug rapidly spreads over, upto margins and easily baths the synovial surface.
4. Patients having affections of the knee, usually present quite early because being a direct weight bearing joint, even mild pain attracts the patient's attention instantaneously. In these stages of presentation, intra-articular injection of corticoid proves, in most of the circumstances, quite effective.

Mode of Injection

The joint can be approached anteriorly or posteriorly. However, anterior approaches being quite easy, are recommended. Anteriorly again, in the infra-patellar region medial or lateral joint spaces are easily negotiable. For the pathology localized mainly, in supra-patellar region; supra-patellar approaches, either from medial or lateral side, can be more helpful.

Infra-patellar Approach

Injection can be given either in sitting or lying down position. Since, in few cases patients are sensitive to local anaesthetics and a few patients are hypersensitive to any prick, it is better to give injections in lying down position.

Lying-down Position (Figure 12.1)

The patient lies supine. The knee is flexed to 60 to 80 degrees. The tip of the index finger can be easily placed over anterior part of upper portion of tibial plateau over which the point of entry should be marked either by skin pencil or nail tip. Thence, after antiseptic preparations, the needle should be pushed backwards, with lateral or medial inclination correspondingly from infromedial or inferolateral compartment, little above and parallel to the tibial plateau, till it is in the joint (which is indicated by loss of any resistance). It must be avoided to push too much within, as it

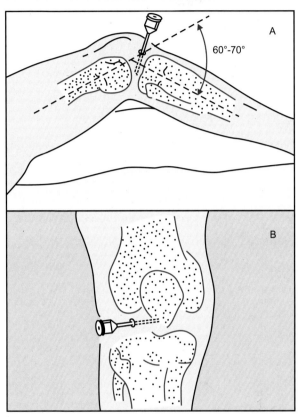

Figure 12.1: Knee joint—Infrapatellar approach in lying down position. Viewed from side (A); from above (B)

may hurt the articular cartilage of femur, whereby the patient feels pain which may persist for a few days with or without swelling.

Supra-patellar Approach (Figure 12.2)

The patient lies supine. Knee is extended and the patient is asked to relax the quadriceps. The patella becomes lax and supra-patellar pouch also becomes loose. Palpate the superolateral or superomedial margin of the patella. Push the needle almost transversly a little above the upper margin of patella with slight upwards and posterior inclination. Try to avoid any contact with the bone. These approaches are usually

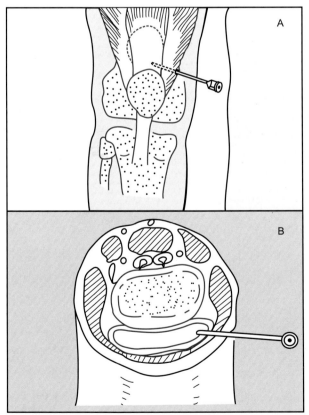

Figure 12.2: Knee joint—suprapatellar approach in lying down position. A—viewed from above; B—section showing needle into suprapatellar pouch

recommended where there is some collection in supra-patellar pouch which makes the thrust of the needle markedly easier into the distended pouch. First, aspirate the collections. Corticoid should be only injected if the aspirate does not appear infected.

Sitting Position (Figure 12.3)

Only infra-patellar injections are recommended in this position. However, supra-patellar pricks can also be made, where there is collection in the supra-patellar pouch. In such cases the knee is extended as far as practicable and the leg is supported over a sandbag placed behind the lower leg. For infra-patellar route, let the patient sit at the edge of the table with the leg hanging or resting on low stool; or on the chair with feet planted on the ground. The knee is flexed at about 90 degree. Locate the upper tibial plateau either laterally or medially and mark it with the nail-edge or skin pencil. After antiseptic cleaning push the needle directly posteriorly, little above and parallel to the tibial plateau with an inclination towards the mid line.

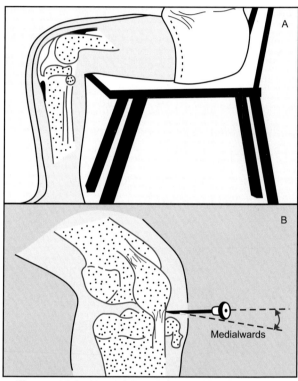

Figure 12.3: Knee joint—infrapatellar approach in sitting position

Posterior Approach

Posterior approaches are usually not recommended for intra-articular injections. In specific conditions e.g. cysts from posterior part of semi-lunar cartilage, capsular cyst, Morrant-Baker cyst or any tendor non-specific condition in relation to posterior part of the knee, corticoid injection may be given by posterior approach. The cyst or spot to be pricked is approached directly, avoiding neurovascular bundle.

The bursae around the knee joint are also treated sometimes by injecting corticoid into them. These are more or less associated with the tendons around the knee joint. Any particular bursa can be palpated in relation to its tendon. It should be clearly delineated first and then pricked by direct approach. It is better to keep the needle inclined parallel to the corresponding tendon.

In the management of the chronic bursitis of the anserinus bursa, infiltration of the corticoid is usually helpful.

Method of Injecting into the Anserinus Bursa

The patient sits at the edge of the table. Palpate the medial side of the tibial crest below the patella. Note the tendinous attachment of the three muscles – [sartorius, gracilis and semitendinosus] – the pes anserinus. The anserinus bursa lies between the pes anserinus and the attachment of the medial collateral ligament of knee at the tibia. The injecting needle is directed parallel to pes anserinus attachment to reach the maximal tender point and swelling.

To further improve the NO TOUCH TECHNIQUE of intra-articular injection the point of injection can be selected visually as follows.

Place the tip of your left index finger on the top of the lateral tibial plateaux. About 0.75 cm above the corresponding point on the medial side of patellar ligament will be the point of inserting the needle on the infero-medial joint space. Similarly place the tip of left index finger on the top of medial tibial plateaux and the corresponding point on the parallel level on the lateral side of patellar ligament, will be the point of inserting the needle into the infra-lateral joint space. Similarly by fixing the patella with index finger the point of injecting on supero-medial and supero-lateral region of patella can be visually fixed.

Corticoid is also used for infiltrating around and/or into the lateral popliteal nerve either for traumatic neuritis or Hansen's neuritis or for entrapment (Figure 12.4A).

The patient lies on the side, with the affected side above, and the knee flexed by about 30 degrees. Palpate lateral popliteal nerve below and behind the head of the fibula where it can be rolled against the neck of the fibula. Fixing the nerve at one point with the index finger, the perineural area is infiltrated with cocktail using a thin (22 bore) needle. The nerve can also be gently injected into, if required.

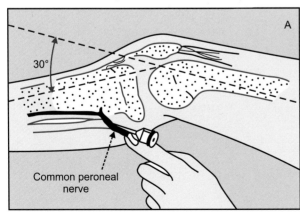

Figure 12.4A: Approach to lateral popliteal nerve

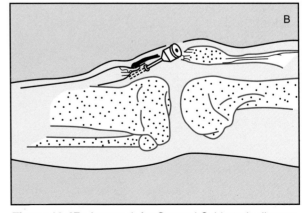

Figure 12.4B: Approach for Osgood-Schlatter's disease

Injection can be given either in lying down position or sitting position. Corticoid cocktail is infiltrated from either side just above the palpable upper limit of tibial tuberosity and just behind the ligamentum patellae. The needle is directed towards mid-line with slight posterior and downward inclination reaching just upto bony resistance (Figure 12.4B).

How to Aspirate Knee Joint?

The patient lies supine with knee slightly flexed (with leg placed on a rolled towel or a sandbag or a small pillow under the popliteal fossa, the patient can comfortably maintain workable degrees of flexion). After thoroughly cleaning and antiseptic preparation, the point of aspiration is visually fixed (not by touching) and infiltrated with the local anaesthesia up to the joint capsule using a long 21 to 22 gauge needle. Then a 18 or 16 gauge aspiration needle is inserted just superior to the upper pole and just lateral to the lateral boarder of the patellae at the level of the patello-femoral joint. The aspiration needle is directed horizontally and at right angles to the long axis of the limb. The needle should enter the joint capsule deep to the quadriceps tendon.

Fluid the joint (most of the fluid remains in the suprapatellar pouch, which is always in continuation of the joint cavity) can be easily aspirated by 20 to 50 ml syringe. However, if there is difficulty in getting the fluid back—perhaps the needle is blocked by a bit of synovium – in such case, release the suction, move the bevel down or slightly in or out and try again. If the fluid initially comes out and then stops, ask the patient to contract quadriceps and slightly flex and extend the knee (most of the patients can do) or ask one assistant to press down on suprapatellar pouch, thereby pushing the fluid into the joint cavity proper and then aspirate. After completing the aspiration take out the needle, put a sterile swab over the puncture-wound, do little massage with finger tip over the punctured zone to block the passage from within and seal the punctured point with tincture of benzoine or povidine iodine.

CHAPTER 13

Ankle Joint

Ankle, on the whole, holds fewer indications for corticoid injection.

Indications

- Traumatic synovitis or arthritis
- Rheumatoid arthritis
- Degenerative arthritis
- Crystal arthritis
- Gouty arthritis
- Ganglion in relation to ankle

Approaches

Approaches are usually anterior. In other sides, the malleoli (medial, lateral and posterior) do overhang the joint to varying extents and hence it is very difficult to negotiate into the joint unless the joint capsule is distended.

Method

1. The patient lies supine. Place a sandbag behind the lower leg. In about 20-30 degree plantar flexed position of the ankle, the anterior joint margin is widened and felt to some extent. Feel the pulsation of anterior tibial artery. Mark a point about a finger breadth on medial side or two fingers breadth on lateral side at which the needle is pushed posteriorly with 20-degree upward inclination. The needle enters without any resistance. Do avoid pricking through a tendon (Figure 13.1).

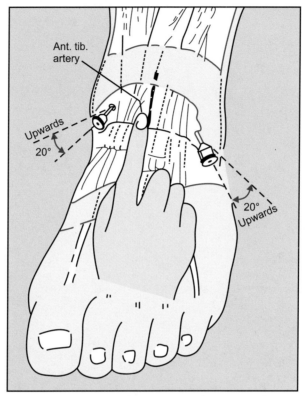

Figure 13.1: Ankle joint—anterior approach

2. The patient lies in the same position as in the above method. Put the index finger just anterior to medial malleolus. With passive movements of the ankle, joint margin can be felt to varying extent, keep that position of the ankle in which the joint space is felt maximum. Push the needle posteriorly with upwards and lateral inclination. Avoid hitting the articular cartilage.

   In the ankle region, tenosynovitis of tibialis posterior and peroneii tendons require corticoid injection. However any tendon in that region can have this pathology.

Tibialis Posterior

It sometimes suffers from non-specific inflammatory changes which often cause pain in that region, that also gets relieved to a varying extent with corticoid injection.

Method (Figure 13.2)

The tibialis posterior tendon stands prominent when patient actively plantar-flexes and inverts the foot simultaneously. The tendon is located above and behind the medial maleollus. Keeping the needle almost parallel to the tendon in that site, it can be pushed upward with a slight lateral and posterior inclination.

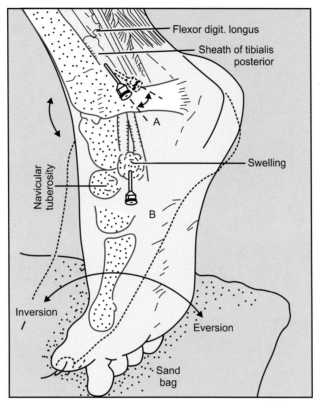

Figure 13.2: (A) Approach to tibialis posterior tendon;
(B) Approach for accessory navicular

The patient lies supine with dorso-lateral aspect of the forefoot supported over a sandbag. The ankle automatically goes in the attitude of plantar flexion and inversion. The needle enters into the sheath, which should be confirmed as follows:

Keep the needle engaged into the supposed sheath. Detach the syringe and ask the patient to relax and then invert the foot repeatedly. With every action of the inversion, the needle moves up and down with tibialis posterior tendon.

Peroneus Longus

Besides tenosynivitis, peroneal spasm leading to spasmodic flat foot also responds to corticoid injection many a times.

Method (Figures 13.3 and 4)

The patient lies supine, keeping his affected lower limb 30 degree flexed and fully internally rotated at hip. The knee is flexed by 30 to 40 degree. This position can be easily held by putting a sandbag beneath the buttock of the affected side. Keep another sandbag beneath the lower leg. Locate the

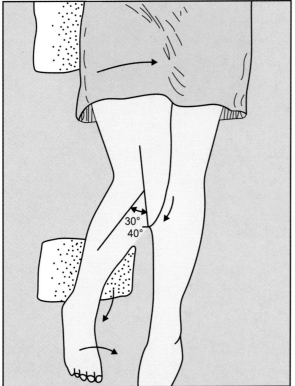

Figure 13.3: Position of patient for injecting into tendon sheath of peroneus longus

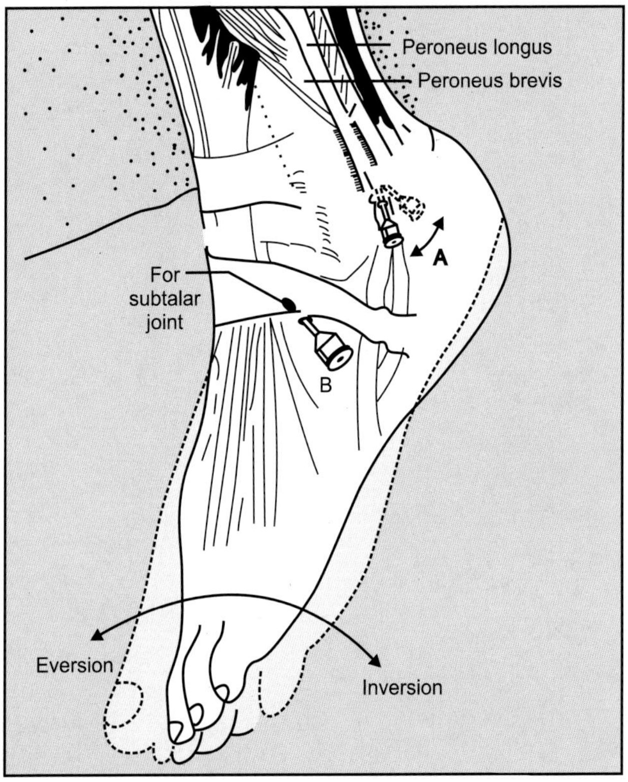

Figure 13.4: (A) Approach to peroneus longus tendon; (B) Approach for subtalar joint

tendon postero-superior to lateral malleolus by asking the patient to plantar-flex and evert the foot simultaneously. Keeping the needle almost parallel to the tendon at the located site, it is pushed posteriorly with upwards and medial inclination. It enters into the sheath. Test by detaching the syringe and asking the patient to actively plantar-flex and evert the foot. With the action of tendon, the needle moves up and down.

Sometimes, ganglions in relation to ankle joint or surrounding tendons are treated by directly injecting corticoid or cocktail.

PAINFUL HEEL SYNDROME (Figure 13.5)

Pain in the heel region has been a common complain due to various reasons. The common conditions requiring corticoid injections are:

1. Pre-Achilles bursitis
2. Post-Achilles bursitis
3. Achilles tendinitis
4. Calcaneal apophysitis

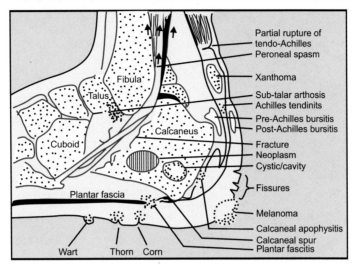

Figure 13.5

5. Plantar fascitis

6. Calcaneal spur syndrome etc.

Non-specific inflammatory conditions around the tendo-Achilles are usually the cause of pain in the back of heel. They may be associated with a swelling of varying consistency in relation to the lowest part of Achilles tendon. Most of the patients present for treatment only when they are symptomatic.

Injection can be given from any side of the tendo-Achilles. The patient lies on the side with mid-leg supported on a sandbag, so that Achilles tendon region remains free from any contact for cleaning from all around. The needle is pushed at a point of maximum tenderness either anteriorly or posteriorly to the tendo-Achilles depending upon whether it is for pre-Achilles or post-Achilles conditions (Figure 13.6).

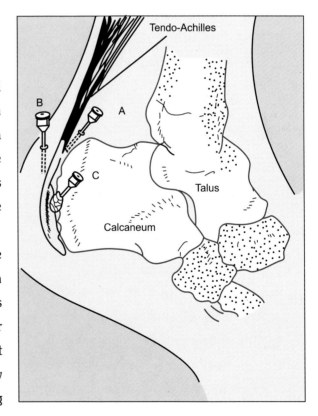

Figure 13.6: Site of injection for (A) Pre-Achilles burisits; (B) Post-Achilles bursitis; (C) Calcaneal apophysitis

In the calcaneal apophysitis (in early adolescent age group) the symptoms are quite often relieved by infiltration of corticoid. The injection should be given into the lowest insertion of tendo-Achilles from either side, better from outer one. The position and method are same as for Achilles-bursitis.

However, boots with raised and softly padded heel top platform should also be recommended alongwith, in such pathologies in and around the Achilles tendon.

PLANTAR FASCITIS

The patient lies supine, with lower leg supported over a sandbag. The leg is kept in externally rotated position (Figure 13.7A). In plantar fascitis, usually the most painful spot is located by pressing with the fingertip towards the under surface of calcaneum on the infero-medial aspect of the sole part of heel at the region from where medial arch takes an upward curve. With a fingertip, this area should be localized by direct pressure. The needle is pushed into the region of maximum tenderness with an inclination backwards, outwards and slightly upwards for about 2.5 cm. Posterior attachment of plantar fascia is usually engaged into, which requires infiltration. By pushing the needle a little outwards the drug can be injected for calceneal spur syndrome (Figure 13.7B).

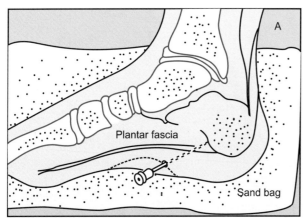

Figure 13.7A: Section showing approach for plantar fascitis

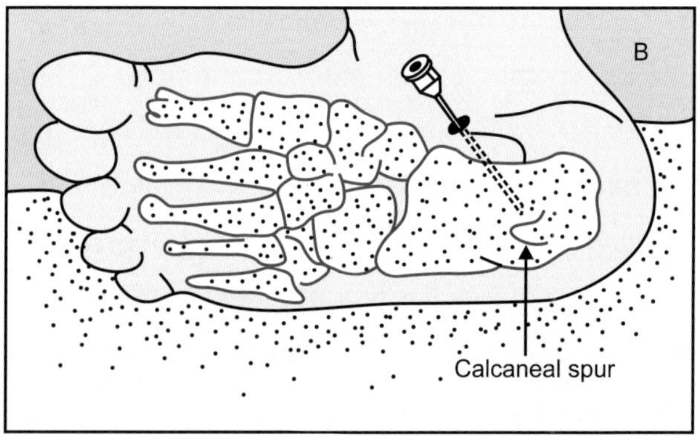

Figure 13.7B: Approach for calcaneal spur

Extracorporeal shock wave therapy (ESWT) is being successfully used for plantar fascitis as well like other orthopaedic indication e.g. lateral epicondylitis. This therapy utilizes shock waves (about 240 per minute) – using electromagnetic shock wave emitter (EMSE) power source vs power source technology – utilizes shock waves which can penetrate even up to 7.5 cm to trigger the body's own repair mechanisms and over-stimulate pain transmission nerves. This therapy is safe, effective and efficient and a high number of shock waves (about 240 per minutes) reduce sensitivity and pain.

Computer-controlled local anaesthetic (or other agents) delivery system (compuMed) is a revolutionary system which allows to easily deliver virtually painfree injection in conditions such as heel spur syndrome, plantar fascitis, neuroma, metatarsalgia, hallux blocks, etc.

Other conditions of foot requiring corticoid injections are:

Symptomatic accessory navicular, bunion in relation to the head of first metatarsal, metatarsalgia, entrapment of 2nd or 3rd interdigital nerves, painful warts, collagen arthropathy, gouty arthritis specially of metatarso-phalangeal and inter-phalangeal joints (in rheumatoid arthritis and gouty arthritis) tendo-vaginitis of tibialis posterior and into peroneal sheath.

Symptomatic Accessory Navicular (see Figure 13.2)

Patient's position will be the same as for injecting into tibialis posterior sheath. Feel navicular tuberosity. Accessory navicular usually lies postero-inferior to it. Infiltrate around this knob-like swelling by direct approach. For osteochondritis of navicular (Kohler's disease) and any other tarsal bone, similar infiltrations around the affected zone work quite satisfactorily and give symptomatic relief.

Subtalar Joint

Following fracture calcaneum, which usually involves subtalar joint in most of the cases, traumatic subtalar arthrosis is a common complication. The patient keeps on feeling pain in subtalar region for 4-5 years, or even more. Usually, walking on the uneven ground or sudden inversion or eversion of foot or keeping foot suddenly on the edge of the step initiates or aggravates the pain. Quite often this condition responds symptomatically to corticoid infiltration.

Method (see Figure 13.4)

Injection can be given with the patient either lying down supine or sitting with foot hanging. It is better with the patient lying down. Patient lies supine with hip flexed 30 degrees and fully internally rotated. The knee is flexed 30 to 40 degrees. The lower leg is supported on a sandbag. The foot has tendency to go for inversion and plantar flexion. Antero-infero-medial to lateral malleolus, the gap of sinus tarsi can be felt. Push the needle directly into the gap medially with slight posterior and upward inclination. The needle enters the region of subtalar joint without any resistance. Also, infiltrate into the sinus tarsi simultaneously.

CHAPTER 14

Spine

In chronic back and neck pain, not amenable to various non-invasive mode of management like, NSAID, postural adjustments, physiotherapy, manipulations, traction, heat therapy, TENSE, inferential therapy etc., injections of steroids (locally in the facet joint, in and around the root, trigger points, etc) may prove useful. In radicular pain locate the desired root, reproduce the pain, block the pain and inject steroid. Generation of trigger spot is mediated through neurogenic impulse and it can behave as an ectopic pain source. Hence, to achieve good result, it is worthwhile to block trigger spots along with the respective root/facet/epidural block. The injection can be given with more precision under the image intensifier. The suspected pain sources should be injected one by one with post-injection clinical assessment done after each injection. Different concentrations of anaesthetic agents (e.g. Xylocain) are used to block different types of neural fibres, such as: 0.5% for sympathetic fibres; 1% for sensory fibres; 2% for motor fibres.

If taken together right from cervical to lumbosacral, the degenerative changes involve the spinal column most frequently. For similar conditions in the limb joints, corticoid injection has been considered as an effective drug for providing symptomatic relief. But, for the spinal joints, this mode of management could not get ground; probably, due to the fact that the joints are comparatively deeply placed and their approaches are circuitous. For conditions like strain, sprain and fibrosistis involving the supra- and inter-spinous ligaments, the corticoids' cocktail injections have been frequently effective. The best guide is to inject at the site of maximum tenderness and the adjoining areas.

Herpetic Neuritis

Corticoid may be effective if injected properly around the involved root. Of course, this is not a very easy procedure. The patient lies on lateral side, with the side to be injected below. One has to use

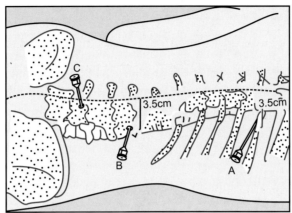

Figures 14.1A to C: Sites of injection. (A) For herpetic neuritis in thoracic region,
(B) For lumbar-disc disease, (C) Intrathecally through LP route

a comparatively long slender needle, and to select the particular root course. Along this course, at about 3.5 cm outside the midspinal line, start with the inclination of the needle up medially and anteriorly along the lower costal margin. Local anaesthetic should be infiltrated first along the course of needle. The moment, proper root is cuffed around by the local anaesthetic agent, the patient's burning sensation and pain will be lessened to a varying extent. Then, the corticoid cocktail is injected at that site and also for some distance while withdrawing the needle (Figure 14.1A).

Lumbar Disc Disease (Figure 14.1B)

In lumbar disc the role of corticoid is variable. It is also not that easy to inject into the disc. This should better be done under the image intensifier. However, in the inflamed state of the disc, help rendered by the corticoid cocktail, either by virtue of producing a dent into the tense discoid space or by anti-inflammatory action is debatable. Further, the inflamed root, if injected appropriately, have been seen to respond well. For prolapsed intervertebral disc, the role of chymopapain has been seen to be more effective, if injected into the disc in earlier stage. Chymopapain, a proteolytic enzyme, can dissolve specifically the nucleus in the intervertebral disc. The process is known as chemonucleolysis. However, this injection must be given by an experienced hand intradiscally under the Image Intensifier.

Anatomy

The epidural space (extradural space, peridural space) is the space between the two layers of the dura mater formed by its division at the edge of the foramen magnum. The outer layer forms like periosteum of the vertebral column and the inner, the actual spinal duramater. The epidural space is limited caudally by the sacrococcygeal ligament. It contains a number of venous plexus as well as fat and connective tissue.

Epidural Steroid Injections

Epidural steroid injections were used to treat local back-pain with associated sciatica since 1950s. Now it has become an integral part of non-surgical management of low back-pain providing relief from one week to one year or even more. On overall assessment about 50% of patients get relief. Caudal epidural can be given through sacral hiatus, interlaminar or transforaminal route.

Principle

The drug, to be effective, must be infiltrated around the affected nerve root.

Indications

- Cases of resistant radiculitis which have not responded to adequate conservative treatment.
- The cases, which have frequent recurrences.
- Annoying persistence of radicular symptoms for pretty long time with fluctuations.

Mode of Injections

Through Sacral Hiatus (Figure 14.2)

The patient lies prone with legs kept extended and with a pillows or sandbag beneath the pubic symphisis. Feel the fused spinous process of sacrum. Slip the index finger gradually down the fused spinous processes. Suddenly, inverted U-shaped deficiency of the sacral hiatus with curved sharp margin on the sides—sacral cornua can be felt. Infiltrate local anaesthetic at the hiatus. After waiting for two minutes (to observe for any reaction and for anaesthetic action), a sterile no: 20 lumbar puncture needle is introduced through the hiatus after holding the skin tight by the thumb and index finger or index and middle fingers of the opposite hand. Straight needle is usually used, but it is preferable to use

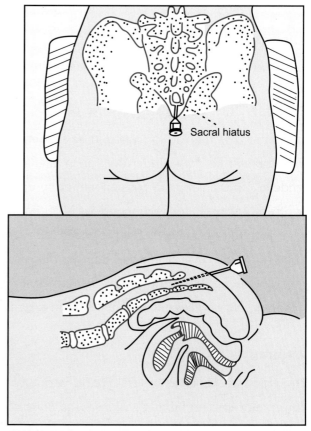

Figure 14.2: Epidural injection through sacral hiatus. Above—viewed from above, Below—sagittal section showing needle in position

bent needle, which facilitates the negotiating of the needle. After negotiating the sacral canal for about 2.5 to 3.5 cm, a feeling of slight yielding can be felt, then stop pushing the needle. Pull the piston of the syringe. If the needle has entered into the epidural space an effortless pulling will be observed and a negative pressure is created in the syringe; and after leaving the piston it returns to the end. The stellate is removed and leakage of cerebrospinal fluid is watched. After confirming that no cerebrospinal fluid was coming out, and there is no resistance in pushing 3 to 5 cc of air within, inject 50 ml of normal saline with 30 to 160 mg of methylprednisolone very slowly. Initially, the patient may feel some pain but very soon it settles down. Let the patient settle down. Again after injecting about 30 to 40 ml of fluid patient feels some bursting pain due to volume injected. Keeping the needle-syringe in situ, pause for a while, the pain settles down. Then complete the injection very slowly. After withdrawing the needle, the patient is asked to turn on side, with the lower limb to which pain was referred lying down. The patient is transferred to bed in lying down position with raised head. The head end of the bed is raised and the patient is advised to rest for 12 hours. Usually, the patient starts feeling better by two to four hours. Usually, one prick is considerably effective, however, depending upon the symptoms, injection may be repeated fortnightly or at monthly intervals. If one injection is totally ineffective, no further injection should be given. It is reasonable to perform up to 3 to 4 injections per year. The patient should take rest on the day of injection. Epidural steroid injection should be combined with usual physiotherapy and rehabilitation programmes.

Through Lumbar Puncture Route (Figure 14.1C)

The patient should lie with the affected side of the root being low. Select the particular space according to the route involvement. Do the lumbar puncture with cautious push so that the subarachnoid space is not entered into, i.e. stop just short of it. After the lumbar puncture needle enters the dura, take out the stylet, connect the syringe. The piston can be pulled effortlessly when the desired subdural space is reached. Inject the local anaesthetic after the appropriate position is reached. If the right position is selected, pain is markedly reduced. Inject 40 to 80 mg of methylprednisolone along with 40 to 50 ml of normal saline. The patient lies for some time (half an hour) in this position.

Injection from the Lumbar Route

Injection can also be given through the lumbar root. The patient lies on the side to be injected below. The course of a particular root is assessed 3.5 cm, outside the midspine line, the needle is pushed, with an inclination upwards, medially and slightly anteriorly to aim at the intervertebral foramina.

Negotiating the needle along the intervertebral foramina corticoid should be injected. Working under image intensifier will markedly facilitate the injection.

Since I Macnab (1971) described the technique of nerve root injection for radioculopathy, it has been found to be effective for radicular pain. Epidural injection of steroids is a popular method for managing lumbar radioculopathy, but has not been commonly used for root injections at thoracic and thoraco-lumbar levels, due to possible neurological complications.

Selective Nerve Root Injection

The term coined by JF Krempen and BS Smith in 1974 has been used diagnostically or to predict the outcome of surgery. Therapeutic efficiency of nerve root injection has been well proved in radicular pain caused by intervertebral disc herniation and discogenic spinal stenosis even to the extent of obviating the need for an operation in more than half of the patients in whom surgery would have been recommended. Nerve-root injections (mixture of 0.5 ml of 2% lidocaine, 0.5 ml of 0.5% bupivicaine and 40 mg of depomedroal) are also effective in the treatment of pain resulting from osteoporotic vertebral fractures. It must be tried in patients with refractory pain from osteoporotic vertebral fractures before considering percutaneous vertebroplasty—percutaneous injection of polymethylmethacrylate (PMMA) into the vertebral bodies to augment the osteoporotic vertebral bodies, or any operative intervention (Don-Jun Kim et al 2003).

Method of Nerve Root Injection

It must be done under the image intensifier. The patient lies prone. After preparing the back skin, the site of the introduction of the needle is localised by the tip of a sterile artery forceps placed at the point of intersection between the lateral margin of the lamina and the inferior margin of the transverse process (as visualised in the fluoroscopy/Image Intensifier). This site of entry is marked with indelible ink. After infiltrating 1% lidocain, a 20-gauge, 13 cm spinal needle is inserted under fluoroscopic guidance into the selected intervertebral foramen. When the nerve root is touched, the patient feels a sharp radiating pain almost reproducing the symptom pain (which he/she was feeling earlier). After confirming by the reproduction of the symptom, the mixture of 0.5 ml of 2% lidocain, 0.5 ml of 0.5% bupivicaine and 40 mg depomedrol is slowly injected.

The injection can be repeated at 2 weeks intervals to a maximum of three or until there was symptomatic improvement. While using nerve-root injection for fractures, too much of steroids must be avoided (maximum of 100 mg).

VERTEBROPLASTY

To augment the grossly (rarefied) osteoporosed painful collapsing vertebrae polymethylmethacrylate (PMMA) is injected percutaneously under the Image Intensifier into the osteoporotic vertebral bodies. The technique is easy and fairly effective in most of the patients in providing relief from pain besides immediate good mechanical results. However, certain possible complications must always be kept in mind such as cell death caused by high polymerisation temperature of PMMA; leakage of PMMA in the adjacent structures; differences in mechanical strength of the injected vertebrae compared with the adjacent ones, etc. Further, the long-term biocompatibility of PMMA is jeopardised by its presence as a permanent implant.

INJECTION INTO AND AROUND THE PERIPHERAL NERVES

Indications are few such as Hansen's neuritis, traumatic adhesion of nerve, early gliosis, entrapment neuropathy (of various nerves at various sites). Common nerves infiltrated are ulnar nerve in and above the medial epicondylar groove; lateral popliteal nerve at and proximal to the neck of fibula; lateral cutaneous nerve of thigh (meralgia paraesthetica) just infero-medial to anterior superior iliac spine.

In entrapment neuropathy, the corticoid cocktail should be injected around the nerve in the compressive canal (fibrosseous or inter-tendinous or inter-musculo-fibrous band).

In Hansen's neuropathy—the corticoid should be injected into and around the affected nerve. Ulnar and lateral popliteal nerves are mostly affected in Hansen's disease, followed by posterior auricular nerve, lateral cutaneous nerve of thigh, etc.

HOW TO INJECT INTO AND AROUND THE ULNAR NERVE

The ulnar nerve is affected in the cubital tunnel and above it on the postero-medial aspect of lower and lower mid-arm—where the tender nerve thickening can be well appreciated.

Method

The patient lies semi-supine with affected side arm externally rotated and elbow flexed by 45 degree. One assistant holds that upper limb by one hand and keeps it steady by holding it at upper part of arm. After preparing from mid-arm to mid-forearm, the needle is introduced around the most palpable ulnar nerve and the prepared corticoid cocktail is infiltrated around the nerve. Then, in case of Hansen's neuritis, the needle is little withdrawn and then gently pushed into the substance of the nerve (easy resistance) and the cocktail is injected. After the needle is withdrawn, the patient is asked to flex and extend the elbow a few time.

HOW TO INJECT INTO AND AROUND THE LATERAL POPLITEAL NERVE

The patient lies semisupinated with the affected side, lower limb flexed at hip by 40 degree and internally rotated by 30 degree and flexed at knee by 45 degree. The lateral popliteal nerve can be palpated and rolled on the outer side of neck of fibula and above it. Injection is made around the nerve at and above the neck of the fibula and into the nerve just proximal to the neck of fibula. After withdrawing the needle, the patient is asked to flex and extend the knee a few times.

HOW TO INJECT AROUND THE LATERAL CUTANEOUS NERVE OF THIGH

The patient lies supine with a thin sandbag placed beneath the hemipelvis on which side the lateral cutaneous nerve of thigh is to be injected. After antiseptic preparation, a point is located, one finger breadth below and medial to the anterior superior iliac spine, in which zone the lateral cutaneous nerve of thigh lies after emerging from beneath the outer end of inguinal ligament. The needle is pushed with upward inclination of about 30 degree at the selected point for about 1 to 1.5 cm depth. The prepared corticoid cocktail is infiltrated in that zone in about 1.5 cm radius. If the injection has been properly given, the patient will have anaesthesia/hypoaesthesia in the palm size area on antero-lateral aspect of thigh in middle and lower 1/3rd junctional zone. However, the patient might have disturbed sensation (hyperasthesia or hypoasthesia) in that zone from beforehand due to entrapment of the lateral cutaneous nerve of thigh.

COMPLICATION OF EPIDURAL INJECTIONS

Locally dural puncture infection and archnoiditis can occur. Preservative free solutions and fluoroscopy should be used to minimise archnoiditis. Systemically, there are certain potential risks of treatment such as decrease in immunity, hyperglycaemia, gastric ulcers, avascular necrosis, etc.

Epidural injections act by inducing steroids directly to the painful root to help in decreasing the inflammation. There may also be flushing effect by removing or flushing out inflammatory proteins causing pain.

COCCYDODYNIA (PAINFUL COCCYX)

For the coccygeal pain without any organic lesion (e.g. due to some pelvic pathology or neoplastic conditions) local infiltration of corticoid cocktail has been observed to be frequently effective.

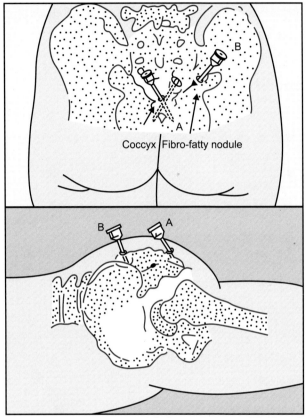

Coccyx | Fibro-fatty nodule

Figures 14.3A and B: Injection for: (A) Coccydodynia, (B) Fibro-fatty nodule:
Above—back view, Below—side view

Method (Figure 14.3A)

A patient lies either in fully prone position with a pillow beneath symphisis pubis or in lateral position. At the lowest end of the sacrum in the natal cleft, the needle is pushed anteriorly with downward inclination, grazing along one margin of the coccyx. The drug is pushed in and around the coccyx as far as practicable. Similar process is repeated on the contralateral side keeping the needle within the skin itself.

In the late cases of subluxation and fracture of coccyx also the above procedure can be adopted. However, in early cases and in acute coccydodynia, injection of long-acting local anaesthetic has been proved to be of more value.

Fibro-Fatty Nodules (Figure 14.3B)

These have been blamed for producing symptoms akin to sciatic radiculitis (pseudosciatica). They usually lie in about upper sacro-iliac zones where they can be rolled under the fingers. Nodules are frequently tender and may trigger the pain down along the course of sciatic nerve. These nodules should be infiltrated into and around by direct approach over it. Depending upon the relief obtained, the corticoid cocktail may be repeated at weekly intervals.

Infiltration into and around Sciatic Nerve

For intractable sciatic radicular pain, injection of local anaesthetic with or without the corticoid, in and around the sciatic nerve in its course through the lower buttock or upper thigh can be helpful.

Method (Figure 14.4)

Along the anatomical course of sciatic nerve, at about the centre of lower gluteal fold, pressing against the femur the sciatic nerve can be rolled or a tendor course of the nerve can be delineated except in fatty patients. Injection should be given directly through a long thin slender needle along the tendor course at any convenient point in and around sciatic nerve.

Old Pelvic Fracture

At times, patients do complain of discomfort and a varying amount of persistent pain in and around the fractured pelvis area, especially the rami. The affected area if palpably tendor, may be infiltrated with corticoid cocktail at weekly intervals.

Recurrent Fibrositis

In recurrent fibrositis either at the root of the neck or anywhere in the span of lumbosacral fascia, local injection of corticoid cocktail often gives a considerable relief.

Rheumatoid Spondylitis

Corticoid injection into sacro-iliac joint gives symptomatic relief in this condition.

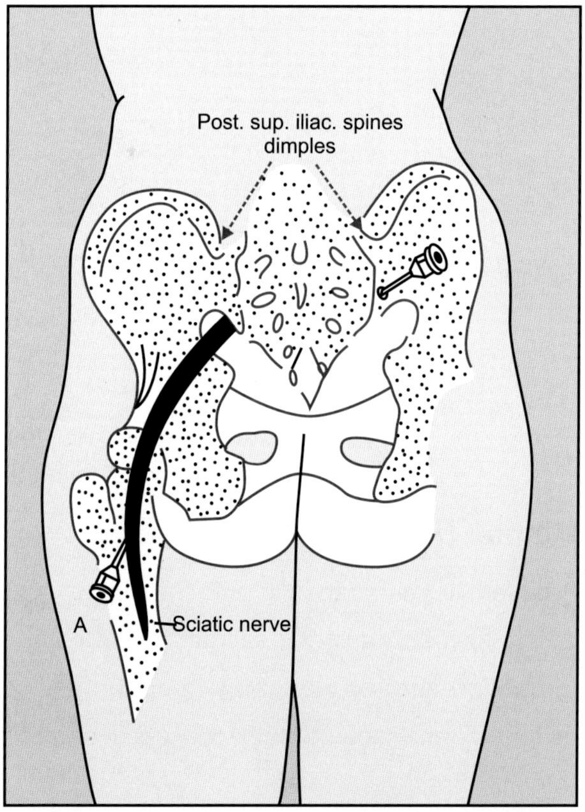

Figure 14.4: (A) Approach to sciatic nerve (in and around), (B) Approach to sacro-iliac joint

SACRO-ILIAC JOINT

Indications

- Sacro-iliac strains and sprains
- Rheumatoid arthritis
- Ankylosing spondylitis
- Unexplained tenderness in the region of sacro-iliac.

Method (Figure 14.4)

The patient lies prone or on the side. Sacro-iliac joints fortunately are represented superficially by obvious dimples. These dimples are more or less superficial to posterior superior iliac spine and adjoining part of upper sacro-iliac joint. These can be easily seen and felt even in obese individuals. The fingertip passing down and posteriorly with slight outer inclination over the posterior part of the iliac crest can easily locate the comparatively rough posterior margin of the joint. Needle should be pushed directly into the joint. Occasionally, the fibro-fatty nodules (responsible for pseudosciatia like condition) also lie in this region. These nodules can also be adequately infiltrated by direct 'touch-feel-inject' technique. In sacral region, indications may be akin to those of the lower spine. In conditions, like fibrotic nodule, fibrofascitis, degenerative conditions, painful spasm in ankylosing spondylitis, rheumatoid arthritis and discitis, corticoid-cocktail injection may have a role, but our experiences in this region have been limited.

CHAPTER 15

Facial Region

In atrophic rhinitis and recurrent allergic rhinitis corticoid infiltration has been found to give relief. This must be done under direct vision using very thin sharp needle working submucously.

Oral Cavity

Post-traumatic or post-infective facial contractures, if infiltrated with corticoid cocktail combined with gradual stretching may yield satisfactory results.

The pale mucosal fibrosis (a rare condition) produces gradual extra-articular ankylosis of the jaw. Since aetiology is not exactly known, the recommended treatment has been empirical. Though difficult to prognosticate, repeated submucosal corticoid infiltration must be tried at bi-weekly intervals combined with gradual stretching of the jaws. In the facial region, temporomandibular joint has been a frequent site for corticoid injection. Common indications are:

1. Fibrous ankylosis of jaw (following rheumatoid, trauma, subdued infection, idiopathic and degenerative arthrosis).
2. Recurrent subluxation of the joint
3. Snapping joint syndrome
4. Postoperative ankylosis of jaw
5. Nonspecific synovitis.

Method (Figure 15.1)

It is better to inject with the patient lying with face turned to opposite side. However, it can also be done in sitting position with head supported on the back of chair. The patient lies down, and face is turned to opposite side as far as possible. Place the fingertip just in front and a little above

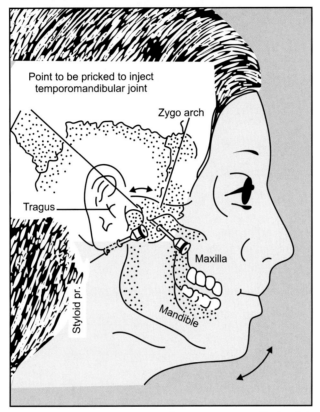

Figure 15.1: Point to approach—temporomandibular joint

the tragus, ask the patient to open and close the mouth frequently. One will be able to feel a gap running antero-posteriorly. While the patient is opening and closing the mouth, judge the position in which the gap is felt maximum. Ask the patient to keep the mouth open to that extent. If he is not cooperative, put a block in the mouth to maintain that position. Through the localised gap, push the thin needle towards midline with slight downward inclination. If it is properly negotiated, loss of resistance will be felt. Repeatedly, confirm by aspiration, for avoiding injury to any vessel, e.g. internal maxillary. Inject a little local anaesthetic and look for any effect in the distribution of facial nerve. At times, any of the branches may be injected, which should be avoided. However, if it happens, its effect will automatically dwindle off within 1 to 2 hours. Inject the corticoid cocktail into the joint. In bilateral cases, the same process can be repeated on contralateral side in the same sitting. Never try to puncture through oral cavity which is dirty, containing numerous organisms.

CHAPTER 16

Joints Around the Clavicle

In painful chronic arthritis conditions, acromio-clavicular joints are also involved. They may require corticoid injection as in other sites. Besides, traumatic synovitis or arthritis can also be the indications.

METHOD

Sterno-Clavicular Joint (Figure 16.1A)

The patient lies supine with a sandbag beneath the neck. Pass the finger medially along the upper border of clavicle. It will terminate into a bony projection. Just medial to it, a very narrow slit can be felt. Push the needle from supero-anterior point of the slit, directly down with little posterior and outwards inclination and infiltrate into the joint. One should avoid going deep lest major vessels may come in the way.

Acromio-Clavicular Joint (Figure 16.1B)

The patient lies supine with scapular region supported on a sandbag. Follow the outer end of clavicle which ends in antero-superior projection. Just outside it a very narrow gap can be felt.

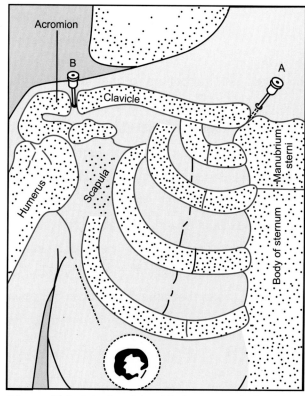

Figure 16.1: Injection into: (A) Sterno-clavicular joint; (B) Acromio-clavicular joint

Push the needle directly into the gap with posterior and a little downward inclination. You are in the joint.

The nonspecific painful conditions with or without swelling of xiphisternum and/or osteochondral junction can also be treated by local injection of corticoid cocktail with varying success. The technique will be more or less one of 'touching, feeling and injecting' the most tendor area.

CHAPTER 17

Occipital Region

In the occipital region there are not many indications for corticoid injection. The tendor fibrotic nodules usually encountered in pressure area or in course of supranuchal line require corticoid injection. Posterior auricular nerve in Hansen's pathology, presenting with thickened nodule may be infiltrated with corticoid cocktail. In the scalp for localised alopecia, keratitis and leucoderma, local infiltration of corticoid has been tried with varying results.

Ophthalmic indications of corticoid are limited. However, in nonspecific keratitis, ocular opacity, fibrotic infiltration of sclera and at times viral ocular palsy, corticoid has been used.

If the facial region, keloids of any region, papillary warts, contact dermatitis and chronic herpetic eruptions may be indications for corticoid injection depending on the clinician's choice.

In Bell's palsy, theoretically, injection of corticoids in and around the stylomastoid foramen may have a local anti-inflammatory action.

Method

The patient lies on the side. In posterior diagastric fossa just behind the neck of mandible, the needle can be pushed, directed medially with downward and posterior inclination taking all possible care of avoiding carotid vessels (by pulsation). Usually the needle tip, if negotiated gradually, hits the bony margin. Pull the needle a little and infiltrate the cocktail.

TRIGEMINAL NEURALGIA

In trigeminal neuralgia corticoid cocktail may give symptomatic relief and sometimes lasting relief to the patients.

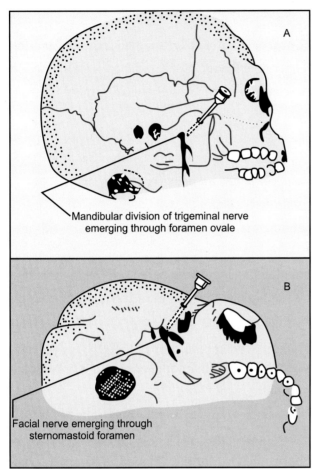

Facial nerve emerging through
sternomastoid foramen

Figure 17.1: In trigeminal neuralgia, corticoid acetate cocktail may give symptomatic relief and some times lasting relief to the patients

Method (Figure 17.1)

Feel the zygomatic notch, and insert the needle 1 cm below it. Advance the tip upwards, backwards and inwards to about 5 cm depth. As the needle tip touches the third division of the trigeminal nerve, the patient experiences severe pain. Local anaesthetic should be injected immediately. The needle point is further advanced. When some resistance is felt, the tip is in the vicinity of the trigeminal ganglion. The corticoid cocktail or 4 ml of absolute alcohol may be injected slowly watching for any side effect simultaneously.

It is difficult to predict the lasting effects of the injection. However, if two consecutive injections are not markedly helpful, it is worthwhile going for resection of the sensory root in the middle cranial fossa.

TRIGEMINAL NEURALGIA

Trigeminal neuralgia, a benign disease, may be defined as short sharp, lancinating paroxysmal unilateral pain in the area of trigeminal nerve distribution.

The disease mainly affects the elderly age group with more incidence in females; however, about 10% of patients are below 40 years of age.

Right side has been seen to be most affected. Usually, the pain appears paroxysmally lasting for a few seconds with free periods in between the attacks. As the disease advances, the number of attacks increases and the free periods become gradually shorter. Ultimately, the pain becomes continuous and agonising which even may push the patient to suicidal point. Any movement of jaws (like chewing, talking, etc), washing of face, exposure to cold wind, etc. precipitates the shooting pain. Usually, a trigger spot develops in the face region, over which even a gentle touch initiates the sudden sharp shooting trigeminal pain.

Aetiology

The exact cause is not known. However, **vascular compression** (usually by superior cerebellar artery or anterior inferior cerebellar artery) at the **TREZ** (**T**rigeminal **R**oot **E**ntry **Z**one) has been blamed for this pain. With the advancing age the arteries become sclerotic and stiff which can cause more pressure.

Other Probable Causes

Idiopathic demyelination of the nerve may result in ephaptic transmission of impulses (i.e. "cross talking" of the axons where in ordinary touch sensation is felt as pain sensation).

In **multiple sclerosis**, sometimes trigeminal pain precipitates.

Tumours in cerebellopontine angle (e.g. meningioma, acoustic, neuroma, epidermoid) may lead to trigeminal neuralgia.

Diagnosis is mainly on typical history. The patient may precipitate the pain by fonding the trigger zone. Objective sensory loss or motor involvement is mainly due to some intracranial organic lesion.

CT scan or MRI is usually normal in idiopathic trigeminal neuralgia; however, only cerebello-pontine angle tumour or other organic lesions can be delineated by CT scan or MRI.

Trigeminal neuralgia can be confused with toothache (where pain is continuous), sphenopalantine neuralgia, atypical facial pain, diabetic cranial neuropathy, glaucoma etc.

Management is medical or surgical—limited invasion; or major intracranial operations, e.g. retromastoid craniotomy and macrovascular decompression. Various medicines (such as carbamazepine phenytain, baclifan, clonazepam, gabapentin, etc.) have been tried with varied degree of success for varied period.

For the refractory patients, other options are:
- Corticoid cocktail injections (see page 68 and 69 for the method injection).
- Peripheral neurectomy
- Rhizolysis with glycerol or radiofrequency lesions, which results in severe dysesthetic pain, which may be sometimes even more worse for the patient.
- Percutaneous trigeminal ganglion balloon compression (PTBC), which is at present perhaps the best choice in percutaneous treatment. Here, under general anaesthesia, a wide-bore needle is passed into the foramen ovale. A balloon catheter is introduced into the Mickel's cave. The balloon is inflated to compress over the preganglionic and ganglionic fibres, which relieves the pain.

It provides long-lasting relief and is suitable for the elderly patients (even complicated with, diabetes, hypertension, coronary artery compromised conditions).

In resistant cases or cases with organic lesions major open-skull surgical operations (e.g retromastoid cranioctomy and macrovascular decompression) may be required.

CHAPTER 18

Complications of Intra-articular Injections

Complications due to Lack of Aseptic Procedure

Mild to moderate, even severe infection (may be associated with features of bacteraemia, pyaemia, septicaemia, even shock) may occur. Unfortunately, this is a common complication. This may even lead to persistent, incapacitating, chronic infection lingering on for years.

1. *Infective arthritis:* It is a major complication which is becoming less, thanks to proper antiseptic care and single-use equipment (syringe tray). It is being estimated at about 1 per 10000, in Western advanced setups. But it still represents a fair number of the arthritis observed in medical practice. It manifests 24 to 36 hours after injection, by intense joint inflammation associated in 50% of cases with hyperthermia. Diagnosis rests on aspiration of joint, cytological examination (highly inflammatory fluid, very rich in altered polynuclear cells) and bacteriologic culture (*Staphylococcus aureus* in 50%).

   How to know the onset of infection

   Usually, after 24 hours of injection, such patients start having increasing swelling and clear inflammatory features (rubor, calor, dolor, tumour, functio laesa), features of cellulitis, pitting oedema, fluctuant accumulation in the joint, even bursting of the abscess and resultant sinus. Constitutional features may accompany to a variable extent, in the earlier phase.

2. *Acute post-infiltrative inflammation:* Microcrystalline arthritis induced by corticosteroids suspensions may manifest in about 5% of the cases. Appearing as acute incident in the early hours following infection (cf-delayed manifestations in sepsis) expressed by a recrudescence of pain with moderate local inflammatory phenomena. The features disappear spontaneously in a few hours; however local application of ice helps.

3. *Tendon ruptures:* Following repeated infiltrations of corticosteroids, rupture of the tendon is not unusual, especially in Achilles heel tendinitis. Intratendinous injection should be avoided as the tendon remains already fragile. The number of infiltrations should be limited in tenosynovitis and tendinitis of the shoulder and elbow.

4. *Destructive "steroid" arthropathy:* Repeated use of local corticoid may produce accelerated destruction of joints; whether due to deleterious action of corticoids on cartilage or cartilage overaction after relief of pain—exact cause is not known. However, if indicated for longer period, interval of prick should be prolonged.

5. *Local skin depigmentation*

6. *Atrophy of cutaneous and subcutaneous tissues:* Repeated infiltration and particularly those of fluorinated cortisone derivatives, (betamethasone, triamcinolone) can produce atrophy of skin and subcutaneous tissue. It has been especially seen in superficial tendinopathies (elbow, wrist, finger region). Hence, in such lesions, prednisolone acetate (3 injections) should be preferred.

7. *Intratendinous and intrabursal precipitate*

8. *General effects of local corticoid therapy:* Though the therapeutic objective of local corticoid infiltration is to avoid the complication of general corticoid therapy, but prolonged local use (for months/years) can induce general side effects (osteoporosis, cataract, cortico-suprarenal insufficiency, probably, due to diffusion even of suspension.

MANAGEMENT OF INFECTION

1. *Prophylactic:* Even with very little doubt in aseptic procedure, it is rewarding to prescribe broad-range antibiotics for 6 to 7 days following the injection.

2. With the earliest features of inflammation, suspect the imminent severe infection and treat it on war-footing with:
   a. Rest to the part either by support or splintage or by traction, as applicable.
   b. Broad-range antibiotics, especially staphylococcal-oriented.
   c. Hot-moist fomentation, 3 to 4 times daily.
   d. Analgesics.
   e. Vitamin B complex and vitamin C.

3. If the features do not start subsiding within 24 hours, there is no harm in putting a wide-bore needle, aspirating the collection, washing the joint with normal saline and injecting antibiotic solution whatever available, pending the result of culture and sensitivity report of the aspirated material. Depending upon the response, the procedure may be repeated even daily combined with suitable antibiotics.

4. Watch the progress. If infection is organising, same procedure may be repeated and continued. If response is not favourable, no time should be lost in performing arthrotomy of the joint, thorough lavage and suitable antibiotic instillation.

   One has to bargain in such circumstances. The infected synovium is a constant source of infection which persists or recurs at intervals. Hence, whenever suspicion exists, synovectomy may be combined in the same sitting. The joint should be closed with continuous closed 'irrigation-suction drainage system', i.e. with the inflowing tube, normal saline with suitable detergent and antibiotic solution is dropped into the joint and through the outflowing tube dirty fluid is drained out.

5. In late cases, with or without sinus, the treatment is the same as that of old septic infections of the joint or other sites. For the joint, ultimately, it may amount to excision-arthrodesis.

6. In very unfortunate circumstances, the infection may persist for pretty long time incapacitating the patient for variable periods. Sometimes the treating team and or the patient gets terribly annoyed of the persistent infection and then one may consider to dispense with the affected part.

For general complications of pyogenic infection, i.e. bacteraemia, pyaemia, septicaemia and shock, the treatment must be on war footing to avoid the hazardous outcome. Besides managing the local infection as above, the possible general complications must be carefully attended from the very beginning—such as:

1. Managing shock.
2. Fluid balance.
3. Suitable antibiotic cover.
4. Electrolyte balance.
5. Blood transfusion, if needed.
6. General build up.
7. Maintaining kidney function and
8. Protein build up.

Complications due to Error on the Part of Clinicians

1. Infections (vide supra)
2. Difficulty or error in selecting the point of injection: In such circumstances, not only the drug does not reach the desired point but it also initiates pain on a site which was hitherto painless.
3. Pushing the needle too deep, so that it strikes the articular cartilage or bony component: Instantaneously the patient feels sharp pain. Subsequently, effusion may appear with increasing

pain. Varying limitations of movements of the joint (spasmodic) may develop. This can be avoided by cautiously pushing the needle into the joint area. However, if it happens, reassurance, cold compress, analgesics, and rest to the part for about two days usually provide marked relief.

4. Sometimes error has been noticed in the materials injected, which can produce complications.

Corticoids can Produce General Complications

- With triamcinolone hexacetonide (THA) injection, hot flushes and facial redness have been observed.
- With methylprednisolone acetate (MPA) also, rarely may be local burning sensation, or rashes.
- Intra-articular injection of bupivacaine and methylprednisolone, there may be anaphylaxis.
- Repeated intra-articular corticoids may lead to local osteonecrosis and marrow fat-induced synovitis.
- Methylprednisolone acetate (MPA) has been observed to provide better response initially for a few weeks.

Complications due to the Drug

As such, anaphylactic reaction and other untoward reactions have been very rarely reported. Hydrocortisone acetate, itself being of corticoid group, is least likely to produce reaction as far as the drug is concerned. Perhaps, reactions noted after hydrocortisone acetate injection might be due to the local anaesthetic used. However, we had occasions to note peculiar reactive changes following intra-articular hydrocortisone acetate injection. Patients started complaining of piercing pain in the joint which showed some amelioration following gentle movement of the joint. Again, after about two hours, they had severe pain in the joint with a sense of exhaustion in the whole body. Thence, a swelling about an inch in diameter appeared on contralateral infrapatellar fossa of the same knee. This was evidenced on both knees in one case where both were injected in the same sitting. General condition of the patients was perfectly all right. They required a good amount of sedative for relief of pain. Such conditions persisted for 18 to 20 hours. Again, whether it was due to hydrocortisone acetate or local anaesthetic, we are not able to say. Sometimes, the patient complains of heaviness in the joint which persists for a day. Whether it is an effect of local prick or due to injected volume of the drug, could not be ascertained. However, this is not a regular phenomenon.

Rebound Phenomenon

It has been noticed that very occasionally the patient gets marked relief of symptoms following even the first prick, but the symptoms reappear with greater magnitude even when the treatment line remains exactly the same and with no features of inflammation. These symptoms do persist for very long periods. No suitable explanation for this bizare manifestation can be offered.

Delayed Manifestations of Infections

Very rarely, we had the occasion of seeing the patients with delayed infection in whom injection was given elsewhere months or years back. The patient presented with subdued features of septic arthritis and we had diagnosed as a case of nonspecific or subacute pyogenic arthritis. When arthrotomy was done, chalky white deposits of previously injected hydrocortisone acetate were noticed, round about which the chronic infiltrative reactive features were also observed.

On histopathological examination, the features of chronic pyogenic arthritis in two cases and chronic nonspecific arthritis in one case were reported. Culture were sterile in all the three cases.

CHAPTER 19

Role of Botulinum Toxin Type A Injection in Spastics

Spasticity results due to insult, injury or damage to either the brain or spinal cord or both (CNS), e.g. cerebral palsy, cerebrovascular accidents, multiple sclerosis, spinal cord injury. Spasticity may be generalised affecting large part of body or it may affect small area such as wrist, hand, ankle (focal spasticity). The severity of spasticity may vary ranging from mild muscle stiffness to severe painful uncontrollable muscle spasm which can affect sitting in a chair or even lying in bed and can make moving from one place or position to another very difficult. Spasticity is almost always a life-long problem. If left neglected it gradually worsens and ends in contractures.

The most important treatment of spasticity is regular physical therapy and relaxing and stretching exercises. Proper treatment of spasticity depends upon the pattern and degree of spasticity. If there is large area affected by spasticity, oral medication or intrathecal medication may be required. If a relatively small area is affected local injection of drugs like phenol or botulinum toxin type A (available as BOTOX) may be given to weaken or paralyse specific overactive muscles. Severe spasticity which cannot be effectively treated with drugs or injections may require surgery. However, physiotherapy and occupational therapy must be continued.

BOTOX (Botulinum Toxin Type A) is a natural purified protein, whose active ingredient is botulinum toxin type A and is extracted from bacteria under controlled laboratory conditions.

MODE OF WORKING OF BOTOX

The electrochemical messages are transmitted from the higher centre to the muscle through the nerves. At the nerve-endings acetylcholine is secreted which initiates the muscular contractions. If due to irratic or abnormal or asynchronus or excessive release of neuromuscular signals too much of acetylcholine is released at the neuromuscular junctions, it induces overactivity in muscular contractions leading to muscle spasm.

Once injected BOTOX binds to the nerve terminal and blocks the release of acetylcholine relaxing overactive muscles. BOTOX temporarily blocks the nerve's ability to release acetylcholine and thus greatly reduces or even stop muscle spasms which relieves the symptoms.

BOTOX has been used since 1989 to treat several conditions presenting with spasticity, especially, in the face e.g. in the management of blepharospasm, neck muscle spasm etc. In blepharospasm BOTOX is given 0.1 ml or less just under the skin and into the muscles around the eye that cause the increased blinking. BOTOX reduces both the strength and frequency of contraction of the eyelid muscles and thus improves the symptoms. The effect lasts for about six months after which injection should be repeated.

In the spastics, the appropriate indication of BOTOX injection is in those where joints can be moved passively and where it is anticipated that weakening of the targeted muscles will not reduce the functional capacity.

BOTOX is injected in the prior-selected muscles which are having spasm with or without pain. The target muscles are identified by using electrical stimulation with the probe attached to the needle passed into the suspected muscle. After confirming the targeted muscle BOTOX is injected into that muscle/s. Small muscle should be injected at 1 to 2 sites, whereas the larger muscles may require 3 to 4 injections (sites). The effect of BOTOX remains more or less confined to the injected muscle only. The injection is like any other intramuscular injection or with little more discomfort. In apprehensive patients local anaesthetic cream or spray may be used.

The effect of BOTOX injection usually starts after a few days with obvious beneficial effect by two weeks. The beneficial effect lasts for about 3 to 4 months, after which muscle starts returning to its pre-injection condition. Proper physiotherapy must be continued while the effect of BOTOX injection is fully available. BOTOX injection can be continued as long as the condition responds to the treatment and does not have any serious allergic reactions or other side effects. However long-term usage of BOTOX can lead to resistance in a patient due to development of antibodies.

There are no serious complications of BOTOX injections. Locally there may variable pain, tenderness and bruising. Rarely there may be symptoms like, joint pain, headache, skin rashes, nausea, dizziness, pruritis, muscle-stiffness, reduced coordination, etc.

CHAPTER 20

Acupuncture

The Chinese have been claiming the immense role of acupuncture and moxybustion for managing several intractable maladies, overall perusal indicates that in orthopaedic arena this Chinese practice has only limited role. Once the bone is grossly involved, the outcome appears limited. However, on face value, acupuncture has been claimed to have symptomatic relief. Su Wen and Ling Shu tried to explain the basic principles of action of acupunctures as to balance the tissue activities, i.e. in case of 'Xu' (deficient activity), apply the 'Bu' (reinforcing method); and in case of 'Shi' (excessive activity), apply the 'Xie' (reducing method).

The fact that the acupuncture analgesia may be mediated through the humoral factors, such as endogenous opoid peptides, has been gaining ground on the basis of recent experimental findings. Low-frequency electropuncture may be mediated in part by beta-endorphins while high frequency electroacupuncture may act through the serotoninergic encephalinergic system.

Moxybustion, based on the principle of the thermal stimulation, perhaps works as a counter-irritant and as a counter-physical stimulant.

As a method of substitute or synergism to hydrocortisone acetate injection into the joints or soft tissues (as discussed in previous chapters), the acupuncture system has some role in low backache, chronic nonspecific arthritis, painful shoulder syndrome, tennis elbow or allied conditions at elbow, de-Quervain's diseases and chronic sprain of lower extremities, especially the ankles. In these conditions too, once gross osteoarticular changes have occurred, the effect of this treatment is not very encouraging. So long as the explanation of the symptoms lies in and around the soft tissues, acupuncture can be an effective alternative tool in the hands of clinicians, especially when the available routine methods have proved ineffective. However, this is a job of an expert and must not be practised by clinicians unless prior practical course has been undergone.

ACUPUNCTURE IN ARTHRITIS

Commonly, rheumatic, rheumatoid and osteoarthritis conditions have been seen being treated in acupuncture clinics. During the acute stage of arthritis treatment should be applied once every day. In the chronic conditions treatment should be given every alternate day. The patient must be asked to undergo physiotherapy simultaneously for quicker recovery.

For low backache acupuncture and/or moxybustion have been frequently tried with, quite often, encouraging results. In acupuncture clinics, patients of sprained lumbar spine, rheumatoid spine, slipped discs, proliferative spondylitis, pelvic inflammatory diseases and even neoplastic conditions have been managed. However, the first three indications are suitable and in rest of the conditions acupuncture can be resorted to as an auxiliary treatment for symptomatic relief. For sprained spine strong stimulation and for muscular strains mild stimulation are given. Acupuncture and moxybustion can be applied simultaneously. Even electroneedling or cupping may also be applied. Treatment is done mainly through selected points, e.g. urinary bladder channels everyday or every other day retaining the needle for 15 to 20 min. After the pain is relieved, the local points are punctured.

ACUPUNCTURE IN PAINFUL SHOULDER SYNDROMES

Conditions like sprain, strain, peripheral nonspecific inflammation, supraspinatus tendinitis, sub-acromial bursitis, biceps tenosynovitis (tendinitis), have been managed by these methods. Fairly strong stimulations are given. Points are selected from the extremities. While manipulating the needle, the patient is asked to exercise the affected shoulder vigorously. Treatment may be given daily or on alternative day.

For tennis elbow, strong stimulations are given at local and distal points.

At the wrist and hand region, de-Quervain's disease, trigger finger and tendon sheath ganglion have been treated by acupuncture with or without moxybustion. Medium to strong stimulation are given daily or every other day. However, corticoid injections, manipulations and surgical treatment have also been recommended as and when needed.

CHAPTER 21

Reiki

"Reiki" is a Japanese word comprising two components.

'Re' = Omnipresent +

'Ki' = Energy of life.

The 'energy of life' comes with life and goes with death.

Dr Mikale Sui of Japan reinnovated the process of 'Reiki'—which had been popular in various forms at least in ancient India. The Saint Guru Vashista (religious teacher and priest of Lord Ram's dynasty) had innovated the process of "Treatment by touch"—**'Sparsh Chikitsha'** which we have forgotten.

The principle of **Reiki** is more or less guided by 'psychosomatic effect'.

They believe that there are seven major energiging points **"Chakra"** in the body, of which four located in the upper part of body are triggered to energige the life.

The Reiki system teaches:
- To control the emotions
- To develop self-confidence
- To undermine the symptoms
- To develop the overall psychological power, strength, will and confidence.

Nonorganic diseases, psycho-oriented diseases/symptoms, depressive psychosis, unexplained symptoms, backache, headache and alike conditions have been claimed to have fastly improved under the process of Reiki.

The process of Reiki can be imparted even in two days. It can be self-imparted as well.

Table 1

S.No. Worker	Year	Materials used for intra-articular injection	Remarks
1. Koning	1932	Iodised oil	
2. Thomson	1933	Pregl's solution of iodine with sodium bicarbonate and Sodium chloride in watery solution.	
3. Key	1933	Claimed to have produced experimental osteoarthritis with intra-articular injection of weak acids, alkalies, distilled water and salt solution. These solutions were later utilised as theraputic measures by Koning Thomson and Andernach	All these were small series with slender theoretical basis and so were denied general acceptance.
4. Andernach & Lohr	1936	Pure liver injections.	
5. Waugh	1936 1938 1945	Lactic acid with procaine at pH 5. He claimed good results in osteoarthritis, traumatic arthritis & rheumatoid arthritis. Discovering the identical pH of synovial fluid to that of blood, i.e. 7.4 to 7.6. Waugh propounded his acidification thereby. He suggested that acidity excites a polymorphonuclear leucocytosis followed later by local metablastic proliferation and this helps in clinical improvement. He further suggested that the change in pH helped to nourish the cartilage better. Acidification theory stimulated other workers who used lactic acid.	
6. Crowe	1944	Acid potassium phosphate(?)	
7. Kron	1948	Sodium bicarbonate	Encouraging results.
8. Lawther	1949	Lactic acid and procaine solution Procaine hydrochloride solution alone	Observed equal results.
9. Melkid	1953	Procaine alone	
10. Ross Mayer & Shepherd	1958	Benzyl salicylate	
11. Desmarais	1952	1. Alkaline procaine solution at pH 7.4 marked difference in these groups. 2. Normal saline pH 7.2 Waugh's acidification theory. 3. Mock injections 4. Waugh's lactic acid, procaine pH 5.4	Did not find any Did not support
12. Baker & Chayen	1948	Lactic acid in 2% procaine (pH 5.4) 0.5% procaine adjusted to pH 7.6 with sodium phosphate normal saline.	The results in the different series were almost identical hence they claimed that acid solution produced no benefit compared to those of physiological pH.

Contd...

Contd...

S.No Worker	Year	Materials used for intra-articular injection	Remarks
13. Scott	1943	10% Benzyl salicylate in oil	Observed good result in osteoarthritis and other rheumatoid disorder.
14. Elkin	1945	10% Benzyl salicylate in oil	Observed encouraging results.
15. Broadman	1954	10% Benzyle salicylate in oil	—Do—
16. Vonreis & Swenson	1951	Osmic acid in animals & painful joint of human beings.	Noticed widespread necrosis of synovium but no effect on articular cartilage. Recommended to be used as chemical synovectomy.
17. Shutkin	1951	Intra-articular nitrogen mustard to effect chemical synovectomy without causing cartilage damage.	Mitchell, Laurin Shepard (1973) contraindicated the utility of osmic acid and nitrogen mustards for effecting chemical synovectomy as these chemicals were subsequently noticed to cause disintegration of cartilage surface.
18. Scherbel, Shuciter & Weyman	1957	Same as (17)	
19. Makin & Robin	1964	Intra-articular radioactive gold for treating chronic synovial effusions.	
20. Chacha, Karim	1978	Intra-articular papain, acetyl salicylic acid indomethacin, prostaglandin and alcohol.	Experimental study to produce a good experimental model of osteoarthritis
21. Thorn (Quoted by Hollander 1951)	1950	Compound 'F' (hydrocortisone)	Intra-articular injection into rheumatoid. Observed encouraging results
22. Hollander, Brown, Jessar & Brown	1951	Compound (F)	Intra-articular injection into inflamed knee, Prompt alleviation of local effect

Contd...

Table 1

Contd...

S.No Worker	Year	Materials used for intra-articular injection	Remarks
23. Freyberg et al (quoted by Hollander et al 1951)	1951	Cortisone	Intra-articular into knee joint.
24. Mason et al (quoted by Hollander 1951)	1951	Preferred hydrocortisone to cortisone for injection.	
25. Miller, White & Morton	1958 1958	To determine the true status of certain intra-articular injections used lactic acid, navocaine hydrocortisone acetate with controls of physiological normal saline and mock injections.	They did not find any significant different series. They suggested the possibilities of physiological implications following injection.
26. Feffer	1965	Intra-discal injection of hydrocortisone in patients having backache. Rest either had no initial response or the patients had presented with recurrences. He inferred that older age group patients having primaerible only backache without any radicular affection and having limited degenerative changes of involved sufficiency well.	47.6% patients responded.
27. Mukherjee K	1982	Acetyl salycylic acid 2% pH 4.4.	Under trial

References

1. Adams ME, Atkinson MH, Lussier AJ et al. The role of viscosupplementation with Hylan G-F 20 (Synvisc) in the treatment of osteoarthritis of the knee: a Canadian multicenter trial comparing hylan G-F 20 alone, Hylan G-F 20 with non-steroidal anti-inflammatory drugs (NSAIDs) and NSAIDs alone. Osteoarthritis Cartilage 1995; 3: 213-25.
2. Andereoh F, Lohr W. ZBI Chir, 1936;63:2493.
3. Baker DM, Chayen MS. Treatment of arthritis, by intra-articular injection. Lancet 1948; 1:93.
4. Balasz EA, Denlinger JL. Viscosupplementation: A new concept in the treatment of osteoarthritis. J Rheumatol 1993; 20(Suppl 39): 3-9.
5. Balazs EA, Bloom GD, Swann DA. Fine structure and gycosaminoglycan content of the surface layer of articular cartilage. Fed Proc 1966;25:1813-1816.
6. Balazs EA, Freeman MI, Kloti R, Meyer-Schwickerath G, Regnault F, Sweeney DB. Hyaluronic acid replacement of vitrous and acqueous humor, 1972.
7. Balazs EA. The physical properties of synovial fluid and the special role of hyaluronic acid. In: Helfet A (Ed): Disorders of the knee. Philadelphia: Lippincott 1974l;61-74.
8. Balazs EA. Viscoelastic properties of hyaluronic acid and biological lubrication. (Symposium: Prognosis for Arthritis: Rheumatology Research Today and Prospects for Tomorrow, Ann Arbor, Michigan, 1967). Univ Mich Med Civ J 1968;(Suppl): 255-59.
9. Barr JD, Barr MS, Lemley TJ et al. Percutaneous vertebroplasty for pain relief and spinal stabilization. Spine 2000; 25:923-8.
10. Broadman J. J Med Sec N J 1954; 51:320.
11. Crowe HW. In Octavio Calvillo, Ioannis Skaribas, Joseph Turnipseed (Eds): Treatment of arthritis with acid potassium phosphate. Lancet 1944;1:563.
12. Desmarais MHL. Value of intra-articular injection in osteoarthritis. Annals of the Rheumatoid Disease 1952; 11:277.
13. Elkin AC. Med Press 1945;213:350.
14. Feffer HL. Therapeutic intra-discal hydrocortisone: A long term evaluation study and analysis. J Bone and Join Surg 1965;47:1287.
15. Friedman DM, Moore ME. The efficacy of intra-articular steroids in osteoarthritis: a double-blind study. J Rheumatol 1980;7:850-6.
16. Gaffney K, Ledingham, Perry JD. Intra-articular triamcinolone hexacetonide in knee osteoarthritis: factors influencing the clinical response. Ann Rheum Dis 1995;54:379-81.
17. Goodman LS, Gilman A. The pharmacological basis of therapeutic (5th edn). New York: Macmillan Publishing Company Inc. 1975;1987-88.
18. Helfet AJ. Management of osteoarthritis of the knee joint. In Helfet (Ed): Disorders of the knee. Philadelphia: JB Lippincott Co 1974;175-194.
19. Hollander JL, Brown Jr, Jessar RA, Brown CY. Hydrocortisone and cortisone injected into arthritic joints. J Arm Med Assn 1951;147:1629.

20. Hollander JL, Jessar RA, Brown EM Jr. Intrasynovial corticosteroid therapy: A decade of use. Bulletin of Rheumatic Diseases 1961;11:239.
21. Hollander JL. Ann Inter Med 1953;39:735.
22. James A, Doherty M et al. Intra-articular corticosteroids are effective in osteoarthritis but there are no clinical predictors of response. Ann Rheum Dis 1996;55:829-832.
23. Jha SS. Observations on the effects of repeated intra-articular injections of hydrocortisone acetate: An experimental study. Thesis for the Master of Surgery (Orthopaedics) Ranchi University, 1978.
24. Karak M, Ugras S, Tosun N et al. The effects of intra-articular administration of hyaluronan and cortisone in the rabbit's knee: A comparative experimental study with histopathologic evaluations. Orthopaedic Update (India) 2001;II(2):68-71.
25. Key JA. Production of chronic arthritis by the injection of weak acids, alkalies, distilled water and salt solution into joints. J Bone & Joint Surgery 1939;15:67.
26. Kim DJ, Yun YH, Wang JM. Nerve-root injections for the relief of pain in patients with osteoporotic vertebral fractures. J Bone Joint Surg 2003;85-B:250-253.
27. Koing W. Zbl Chir 1930;59:1907.
28. Kron R. Die intra-articular-alkali—Therapic schweizer ische medizinesche wochenschrift 1948;78:80.
29. Lawther K. Ann Rheum Dis 1948;8:178.
30. Makin M, Robin GC. Chronic synovial effusions treated with intra-articular radioactive gold. J American Medical Association 1964;188:725.
31. Melkid A. None Erfaringer Med procainbe handling Tidaskrift for den Norske Laegefor 1953; 73:484.
32. Miller JH, White J, Morton TH. The value of intra-articular injections in osteoarthritis of the knee. J Bone and Joint Surg 1958;403:636.
33. Namiki O, Toyoshima H, Morisaki N, Watnabe Y, Yamaguchi T. Studies on some properties of synovial fluid. Orthop Res Science 1978;5:163-168.
34. Natarajan M: Trigeminal neuralgia-percutaneous trigeminal ganglion balloon compression. In hand bulletin of KG hospital, Coimbatore.
35. Octavio Calvillo, Ioannis Skaribas, Joseph Turnipseed. Anatomy and pathophysiology of the sacroiliac joint: Current Review of PAIN-(official publicator Lalorld Inscitute of Pain). Philadelphia: Current Science Inc. Panther Publishers Private Limited, Bangalore 2001;12 to 17.
36. Poro MA, Balasz EA, Belmote. Reduction of sensory responses to passive movements of inflamed knee joints by Hylan, a hyaluronan derivative. Exp Brain Res 1997;Hb: 3-9.
37. Raynauld JP, Buckland-Wright C, Ward R et al. Safety and efficacy of intra-articular steroid injections on the progression of knee osteoarthritis: a randomized double-bind, placebo-controlled trial. Arthritis Rheum 2003;48:370-7.
38. Raynauld JP. Clinical trials: Impact of intra-articular steroid injections on the progression of knee osteoarthritis. Osteoarthritis Cartilage 1999;7:348-9.
39. Ross KA, Mayer JH, Shepher MM. Osteoarthritis of the knee. Treatment by local injection of salicylate compounds. British Medical Journal 1958;1:1040.
40. Scherbel AL, Schueter SL, Weyman SJ. A rotational approach to the treatment of rheumatoid arthritis. Cleveland Clinic Quarterly 1957;24:78.
41. Scott GL. British Med J 1943;2:510.
42. Shutkin NM. Note on the use of nitrogen mustard in rheumatoid arthritis. J Bone and Joint Surg 1951;33:265.
43. Thomson JEM. Biophysical Journal 1933;15:483.
44. Waugh WC. Treatment of certain joint lesions by injection of lactic acid. Lancet 1938;1:487.
45. Waugh WG. Mono-articular osteoarthritis of the hip. British Medical Journal 1945;1:873.

Index